Mild Cognitive Impairment

Editors

BIRJU B. PATEL
N. WILSON HOLLAND

CLINICS IN GERIATRIC MEDICINE

www.geriatric.theclinics.com

November 2013 • Volume 29 • Number 4

ELSEVIER

1600 John F. Kennedy Boulevard • Suite 1800 • Philadelphia, Pennsylvania, 19103-2899

http://www.theclinics.com

CLINICS IN GERIATRIC MEDICINE Volume 29, Number 4
November 2013 ISSN 0749-0690, ISBN-13: 978-0-323-24223-3

Editor: Yonah Korngold

Clinics in Geriatric Medicine (ISSN 0749-0690) is published quarterly by Elsevier Inc., 360 Park Avenue South, New York, NY 10010-1710. Months of issue are February, May, August, and November. Business and Editorial Offices: 1600 John F. Kennedy Blvd., Suite 1800, Philadelphia, PA 191023-2899. Periodicals postage paid at New York, NY, and additional mailing offices. Subscription prices are $269.00 per year (US individuals), $475.00 per year (US institutions), $137.00 per year (US student/resident), $350.00 per year (Canadian individuals), $591.00 per year (Canadian institutions), $186.00 per year (Canadian student/resident), $372.00 per year (foreign individuals), $591.00 per year (foreign institutions), and $186.00 per year (foreign student/resident). Foreign air speed delivery is included in all *Clinics* subscription prices. All prices are subject to change without notice. POSTMASTER: Send address changes to *Clinics in Geriatric Medicine*, Elsevier Health Sciences Division, Subscription Customer Service, 3251 Riverport Lane, Maryland Heights, MO 63043. Telephone: 1-800-654-2452 (U.S. and Canada); 314-447-8871 (outside U.S. and Canada). Fax: 314-447-8029. E-mail: journalscustomerservice-usa@elsevier.com (for print support) or journalsonlinesupport-usa@elsevier.com (for online support).

Reprints. For copies of 100 or more, of articles in this publication, please contact the Commercial Reprints Department, Elsevier Inc., 360 Park Avenue South, New York, New York 10010-1710. Tel.: 212-633-3874; Fax: 212-633-3820, email: reprints@elsevier.com.

Clinics in Geriatric Medicine is covered in *MEDLINE/PubMed (Index Medicus)*, *EMBASE/Excerpta Medica, Current Contents/Clinical Medicine (CC/CM)*, and the *Cumulative Index to Nursing & Allied Health Literature.*

Printed and bound by CPI Group (UK) Ltd, Croydon, CR0 4YY

Transferred to digital print 2012

Contributors

EDITORS

BIRJU B. PATEL, MD, FACP, AGSF
Assistant Professor of Medicine, Division of General Medicine and Geriatrics, Emory University School of Medicine; Director of the Mild Cognitive Impairment Clinic, Atlanta Veterans Affairs Medical Center, Atlanta, Georgia

N. WILSON HOLLAND, MD, FACP
Associate Professor of Medicine, Division of General Medicine and Geriatrics, Department of Medicine, Emory University School of Medicine, Atlanta Veterans Affairs Medical Center, Atlanta, Georgia

AUTHORS

BENJAMIN A. BENSADON, EdM, PhD
Adjunct Instructor, Donald W. Reynolds Department of Geriatric Medicine, University of Oklahoma Health Sciences Center, Oklahoma City, Oklahoma

MALAZ A. BOUSTANI, MD, MPH
Associate Professor, Indiana University Center for Aging Research; Regenstrief Institute, Inc; Department of Medicine, Indiana University School of Medicine, Indianapolis, Indiana

GREGORY S. BROWN, MA
Department of Rehabilitation Medicine, Emory University, Atlanta, Georgia

NOLL L. CAMPBELL, PharmD
Research Assistant Professor, College of Pharmacy, Purdue University, West Lafayette; Indiana University Center for Aging Research, Indianapolis; Regenstrief Institute, Inc; Department of Pharmacy, Wishard/Eskenazi Health Services, Indianapolis, Indiana

DONALD L. COURTNEY, MD
Staff Physician, Section of Geriatric Medicine (11G), Associate Professor, Division of General and Geriatric Medicine, Department of Medicine, Ralph H. Johnson VA Medical Center, Medical University of South Carolina, Charleston, South Carolina

BENJAMIN M. HAMPSTEAD, PhD
Research Clinical Neuropsychologist, Rehabilitation R&D Center of Excellence, Atlanta VAMC, Decatur; Assistant Professor, Department of Rehabilitation Medicine, Emory University, Atlanta, Georgia

CAROLINE N. HARADA, MD
Investigator, Geriatrics Research, Education, and Clinical Center, Birmingham Veterans Affairs Medical Center; Associate Professor of Medicine, Division of Gerontology, Geriatrics, and Palliative Care, University of Alabama at Birmingham, Birmingham, Alabama

BABAR A. KHAN, MD, MS
Assistant Professor, Indiana University Center for Aging Research; Regenstrief Institute, Inc; Department of Medicine, Indiana University School of Medicine, Indianapolis, Indiana

DAVID S. KNOPMAN, MD
Department of Neurology, Mayo Clinic, Rochester, Minnesota

MICHAEL A. LAMANTIA, MD, MPH
Assistant Professor, Indiana University Center for Aging Research; Regenstrief Institute, Inc; Department of Medicine, Indiana University School of Medicine, Indianapolis, Indiana

J. RILEY MCCARTEN, MD
Associate Professor, Department of Neurology, University of Minnesota Medical School; Medical Director, Geriatric Research, Education and Clinical Center (GRECC), Veterans Affairs Health Care System, Minneapolis, Minnesota

MARISSA C. NATELSON LOVE, MD
Instructor/Fellow, Division of Memory Disorders and Behavioral Neurology, Department of Neurology, University of Alabama at Birmingham, Birmingham, Alabama

GERMAINE L. ODENHEIMER, MD
Associate Professor, Donald W. Reynolds Department of Geriatric Medicine, University of Oklahoma Health Sciences Center, and Oklahoma City VA Medical Center, Oklahoma City, Oklahoma

SUZANNE PENNA, PhD, ABPP
Assistant Professor, Department of Rehabilitation Medicine, Emory University School of Medicine, Center for Rehabilitation Medicine; Atlanta Veteran's Affairs Medical Center, Atlanta, Georgia

RONALD C. PETERSEN, MD, PhD
Cora Kanow Professor of Alzheimer's Disease Research, Division of Behavioral Neurology, Department of Neurology, Director, Mayo Alzheimer's Disease Research Center, Mayo Clinic, Rochester, Minnesota

ROSEBUD ROBERTS, MS, MB ChB
Division of Epidemiology, Department of Health Sciences Research; Department of Neurology, Mayo Clinic, Rochester, Minnesota

KRISTEN L. TRIEBEL, PsyD
Assistant Professor of Neurology, Department of Neurology, University of Alabama at Birmingham, Birmingham, Alabama

FRED UNVERZAGT, PhD
Professor, Department of Psychiatry, Indiana University School of Medicine, Indianapolis, Indiana

MEREDITH WICKLUND, MD
Fellow, Division of Behavioral Neurology, Department of Neurology, Mayo Clinic, Rochester, Minnesota

Contents

therefore, is indispensable. Evaluating cognitive symptoms requires a deliberate approach to define the onset, course, and nature of symptoms. An informant who knows the patient well is essential. The physician must have a working knowledge of the basics of cognitive function. The neurologic examination also is fundamental to defining the origin of cognitive impairment. Extraocular movements, speech, and gait are examples of high-yield examination findings that can be observed and tested quickly, adding to the clinical impression.

Knowledge of aging and dementia is rapidly evolving with the aim of identifying individuals in the earliest stages of disease processes. Biomarkers allow clinicians to show the presence of a pathologic process and resultant synapse dysfunction and neurodegeneration, even in the earliest stages. This article focuses on biomarkers for mild cognitive impairment caused by Alzheimer disease, structural magnetic resonance imaging, fluorodeoxyglucose positron emission tomography (PET) or single-photon emission computed tomography, and PET with dopamine ligands. Although these biomarkers are useful, several limitations exist. Several new biomarkers are emerging and a more biological characterization of underlying pathophysiologic spectra may become possible.

Advances in structural and functional neuroimaging techniques have unquestionably improved understanding of the development and progression of Alzheimer disease (AD), with evidence supporting regional (and network) change that underlies cognitive decline across the "healthy" aging/mild cognitive impairment (MCI)/AD spectrum. This review focuses on visual rating scales and volumetric analyses that could be easily integrated into clinical practice, followed by a review of functional neuroimaging findings suggesting that widespread cerebral dysfunction underlies the learning and memory deficits in MCI. Evidence of preserved neuroplasticity in this population and that cognitive rehabilitation techniques may capitalize on this plasticity to improve cognition in those with MCI is also discussed.

Efforts toward early detection of Alzheimer disease (AD) have focused on refinement and identification of diagnostic markers, with the goal of preventing or delaying disease progression. Mild cognitive impairment (MCI) has emerged as a potential precursor to dementia. Though not without controversy, MCI has been associated with an increased risk for conversion to AD. In this article, with emphasis on meta-analyses, randomized controlled trials, and extant literature reviews, considerations and recommendations for optimal clinical management of MCI are offered. Given the substantial heterogeneity of this patient population and inconsistent research methodologies, the need for informed, clinical judgment is critical.

The increasing prevalence of cognitive impairment among the older adult population warrants attention to the identification of practices that may minimize the progression of early forms of cognitive impairment, including the transitional stage of mild cognitive impairment (MCI), to permanent stages of dementia. This article identifies both markers of disease progress and risk factors linked to the progression of MCI to dementia. Potentially modifiable risk factors may offer researchers a point of intervention to modify the effect of the risk factor and to minimize the future burden of dementia.

Mild cognitive impairment (MCI) is a unique entity in the spectrum of syndromes of cognitive loss. Many patients referred for evaluation of memory loss come with an assumption that they already have dementia. When patients are diagnosed with MCI, they and their caregivers have to deal with the challenge of uncertainties. Patient and family education must stress the uncertainty of whether the deficits will progress. This article aims to guide the clinician who has reached a diagnosis of MCI and is working with the patient and family on coping with the uncertainties of MCI.

CLINICS IN GERIATRIC MEDICINE

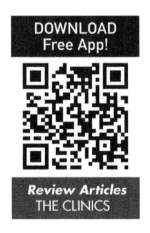

Preface

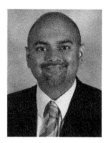 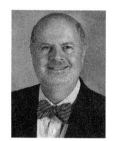

Birju B. Patel, MD, FACP, AGSF   N. Wilson Holland, MD, FACP
Editors

Mild Cognitive Impairment (MCI) is a concept that is very useful and worthwhile in terms of recognition of early cognitive deficits and the earliest stage of possible intervention and planning for the future. From the first time the term was used in 1997 by the Mayo Clinic group headed by Dr Ronald Petersen[1] to the most recent iteration of the definition by the National Institute on Aging and Alzheimer's Association workgroup,[2] there has been an a great deal of thought and research on the topic. In 2010, more than 1220 publications listed MCI in the title, abstract, or key words (Elsevier SciVerse Scopus). Interest in this condition continues to grow along with a rise in the geriatric population, which some term as "the silver tsunami." Not until very recently did MCI get its own official diagnostic code, allowing physicians to bill insurers for reimbursement, thus raising the importance of separating it as a unique entity.

There is still a great deal we do not know about MCI. In this edition, a number of key topic areas at the forefront of MCI are reviewed. Dr Harada and coworkers review aging and cognition, describing how normal aging influences cognitive abilities. It is very important to understand normal to be able to distinguish abnormal. Dr Roberts reviews the epidemiology and challenges in defining MCI. Dr Penna discusses the common symptoms, manifestations, and neuropsychology of MCI. Dr McCarten's review of evaluating early cognitive concerns sets up a clinical framework for busy clinicians in important aspects and foci in terms of evaluation. This is a neurologist's perspective but written for generalists as well. Biomarkers in cognition are reviewed by Drs Wicklund and Petersen. Dr Hampstead and colleagues summarize imaging modalities in evaluating cognitive concerns. Both topics, biomarkers and imaging, bring the reader to the forefront of a large body of research in these fields. Managing MCI is very challenging and Drs Bensadon and Odenheimer shed light in their review on a good approach of "hope for the best, plan for the worst." Progression from MCI to dementia is an area of great unknowns and this topic is laid out clearly in this issue by Dr Campbell and coworkers with current evidence-based summaries. This is something that patients and family members are always curious to know and the concern frequently is brought up to clinicians. Dr Courtney focuses on the topic of dealing with the diagnosis for patients and caregivers. This is dealt with in a patient-centered

Clin Geriatr Med 29 (2013) ix–x
http://dx.doi.org/10.1016/j.cger.2013.07.001
0749-0690/13/$ – see front matter © 2013 Published by Elsevier Inc.

manner with questions that patients and family members have and resources and evidence that exist.

Overall, we are proud to bring you this issue focusing on Mild Cognitive Impairment written by experts in the field highlighting important aspects and topics. MCI will remain a challenge as the population ages and the health care system deals with the economic costs of caring for patients with cognitive impairment and dementia.

Birju B. Patel, MD, FACP, AGSF
Assistant Professor of Medicine
Division of General Medicine and Geriatrics
Emory University School of Medicine
Director of the Mild Cognitive Impairment Clinic
Atlanta Veterans Affairs Medical Center
Atlanta, Georgia

N. Wilson Holland, MD, FACP
Associate Professor of Medicine
Division of General Medicine and Geriatrics
Department of Medicine
Emory University School of Medicine
Atlanta Veterans Affairs Medical Center
Atlanta, Georgia

E-mail addresses:
gerimd@gmail.com (B.B. Patel)
Wilson.Holland@va.gov (N.W. Holland)

REFERENCES

1. Petersen RC, Smith GE, Waring SC, et al. Aging, memory, and mild cognitive impairment. Int Psychogeriatr 1997;9(Suppl 1):65–9.
2. Albert MS, DeKosky ST, Dickson D, et al. The diagnosis of mild cognitive impairment due to Alzheimer's disease: recommendations from the National Institute on Aging–Alzheimer's Association workgroups on diagnostic guidelines for Alzheimer's disease. Alzheimers Dement 2011;7(3):270–9.

Normal Cognitive Aging

Caroline N. Harada, MD[a,*], Marissa C. Natelson Love, MD[b],
Kristen L. Triebel, PsyD[c]

KEYWORDS

- Mild cognitive impairment • Dementia • Aging • Cognition

KEY POINTS

- The normal aging process is associated with declines in certain cognitive abilities, such as processing speed and some aspects of memory, language, visuospatial function, and executive function.
- Although these declines are as yet not well understood, promising developments in neurology research have identified declines in volume of gray and white matter and changes in white matter function that may contribute to observed cognitive changes with aging.
- These changes are small and should not result in impairment in function; nonetheless, driving and certain other activities may be compromised, and it is important to detect safety issues early.
- Participation in certain activities, building cognitive reserve, and engaging in cognitive retraining are all potential approaches to achieving successful cognitive aging.
- The majority of adults older than 65 years will develop neither dementia nor mild cognitive impairment, and more work is needed to better understand normal cognitive aging so that quality of life for these individuals can be maximized.

INTRODUCTION

The number of Americans older than 65 years is projected to more than double in the next 40 years, increasing from 40.2 million in 2010 to 88.5 million in 2050.[1] It will become increasingly important to understand the cognitive changes that accompany

Funding Sources: Dr Harada, Donald W. Reynolds Foundation; Dr Natelson Love, None; Dr Triebel, NIH KL2TR000166: Triebel, PI.
Conflict of Interest: None.
[a] Geriatrics Research, Education, and Clinical Center, Birmingham Veterans Affairs Medical Center; Division of Gerontology, Geriatrics, and Palliative Care, University of Alabama at Birmingham, CH-19-201, 1720 Second Avenue South, Birmingham, AL 35294, USA; [b] Division of Memory Disorders and Behavioral Neurology, Department of Neurology, University of Alabama at Birmingham, Sparks Center, Suite 620D, 1720 7th Avenue South, Birmingham, AL 35233, USA; [c] Department of Neurology, University of Alabama at Birmingham, Sparks Center, Suite 650, 1720 7th Avenue South, Birmingham, AL 35294-0017, USA
* Corresponding author.
E-mail address: charada@uabmc.edu

aging, both normal and pathologic. Although dementia and mild cognitive impairment are both common, even those who do not experience these conditions may experience subtle cognitive changes associated with aging. These normal cognitive changes are important to understand because, first, they can affect an older adult's day-to-day functioning, and second, they can help distinguish normal from disease states. This article first describes the neurocognitive changes observed in normal aging, followed by a description of the structural and functional alterations seen in aging brains that may explain observed cognitive changes. After discussing some of the practical implications of normal cognitive aging, the article concludes with a discussion of what is known about factors that may mitigate age-associated cognitive decline.

METHODOLOGICAL ISSUES WITH STUDIES OF BRAIN AGING

Before discussing normal age-related changes, it is necessary to mention a few common methodological challenges that plague the study of normal brain aging. As with all studies of aging, selection bias is a challenge. Many potential study participants decline enrollment because they are either too healthy (and busy) or too ill.[2] In addition, people with limited social or financial support and functional limitations may be less likely to enroll in studies.[3] This shortcoming results in study findings that may not be generalizable to all older adults.

Because results can be generated more quickly, most studies rely on cross-sectional design, comparing subjects from different age groups.[4] However, such studies are subject to confounding because of cohort differences. A cohort that was born in the 1920s had a life experience very different to a cohort born in the 1980s. These cohorts may differ greatly in terms of culture, lifestyle, education, and requirements for success in life. Subjects from one age cohort may perform very poorly on any given cognitive or neurologic test compared with subjects from a different age cohort irrespective of cognitive capacity, simply because of vastly different life experiences and skill sets.[5] Cohort differences can confound cross-sectional studies by potentially overestimating the effects of aging.[6]

Longitudinal studies are likely better, but these studies also are subject to bias. Study populations will undergo attrition over time, and because those subjects who are most likely to remain in the study tend to be the healthiest, best educated, wealthiest, and have the highest scores on cognitive tests at baseline, the study findings may cease to represent the original study group.[7] Longitudinal studies of cognition also are subject to practice effects: because subjects are required to repeat the same tests multiple times, they may be able to improve or maintain their test scores despite a cognitive decline.[8,9]

Finally, studies of "normal" aging can be complicated when subjects are misdiagnosed as cognitively normal during study enrollment or when subjects develop cognitive impairment during the course of the study. This problem is a concern because dementia onset tends to be insidious, and early symptoms can be easily missed.[4,10]

NEUROCOGNITIVE CHANGES IN AGING

Cognitive change as a normal process of aging has been well documented in the scientific literature. Some cognitive abilities, such as vocabulary, are resilient to brain aging and may even improve with age. Other abilities, such as conceptual reasoning, memory, and processing speed, decline gradually over time. There is significant heterogeneity among older adults in the rate of decline in some abilities, such as measures of perceptual reasoning and processing speed.[11] Here a brief overview of the current neuropsychology of normal cognitive aging is provided. Interested readers are directed to other sources for a more comprehensive review of this topic.[4,12]

Crystallized and Fluid Intelligence

Concepts of crystallized and fluid intelligence are used to describe patterns of cognitive change over the life span. Crystallized intelligence refers to skills, ability, and knowledge that is overlearned, well-practiced, and familiar.[4] Vocabulary and general knowledge are examples of crystallized abilities. Crystallized abilities remain stable or gradually improve at a rate of 0.02 to 0.003 standard deviations per year through the sixth and seventh decades of life.[13] Because crystallized intelligence is due to accumulation of information based on one's life experiences, older adults tend to perform better at tasks requiring this type of intelligence when compared with younger adults. By contrast, fluid intelligence refers to abilities involving problem-solving and reasoning about things that are less familiar and are independent of what one has learned. Fluid cognition includes a person's innate ability to process and learn new information, solve problems, and attend to and manipulate one's environment.[14] Executive function, processing speed, memory, and psychomotor ability are considered fluid cognitive domains. Many fluid cognitive abilities, especially psychomotor ability and processing speed, peak in the third decade of life and then decline at an estimated rate of −0.02 standard deviations per year.[13]

Cognitive ability can be divided into specific cognitive domains including processing speed, attention, memory, language, visuospatial abilities, and executive functioning/reasoning.

Processing Speed

Processing speed refers to the speed with which cognitive activities are performed as well as the speed of motor responses. This fluid ability begins to decline in the third decade of life and continues to decline throughout the life span.[12,15,16] Many of the cognitive changes reported in healthy older adults are the result of slowed processing speed. This "slowing" can negatively affect performance on many neuropsychological tests designed to measure other cognitive domains (eg, verbal fluency). Thus, a decline in processing speed can have implications across a variety of cognitive domains.

Attention

Attention refers to the ability to concentrate and focus on specific stimuli. Simple auditory attention span (also known as immediate memory) as measured by repetition of a string of digits shows only a slight decline in late life.[4] A more noticeable effect of age is seen on more complex attention tasks, such as selective and divided attention.[15,16] Selective attention is the ability to focus on specific information in the environment while ignoring irrelevant information. Selective attention is important for tasks such as engaging in a conversation in a noisy environment or driving a car. Divided attention is the ability to focus on multiple tasks simultaneously, such as talking on the phone while preparing a meal. Older adults also perform worse than younger adults on tasks involving working memory,[17] which refers to the ability to momentarily hold information in memory while simultaneously manipulating such information. For example, older adults may have difficulty ordering a string of letters and numbers in the correct alphanumerical sequence, or calculating a tip on a restaurant bill.

Memory

One of the most common cognitive complaints among older adults is change in memory. Indeed, as a group, older adults do not perform as well as younger adults on a variety of learning and memory tests. Age-related memory changes may be related to slowed processing speed,[18] reduced ability to ignore irrelevant information,[19] and decreased use of strategies to improve learning and memory.[20,21]

Two major types of memory are declarative and nondeclarative memory. Declarative (explicit) memory is conscious recollection of facts and events. Two types of declarative memory include semantic memory and episodic memory. Semantic memory involves fund of information, language usage, and practical knowledge; for example, knowing the meaning of words. Episodic memory (also known as autobiographical memory) is memory for personally experienced events that occur at a specific place and time. Episodic memory can be measured by memory of stories, word lists, or figures. While declines in semantic and episodic memory occur with normal aging, the timing of these declines is different. Episodic memory shows lifelong declines, whereas semantic memory shows a decline in late life.[22]

Nondeclarative (implicit) memory is the other major type of memory, and exists outside of a person's awareness. An example of implicit memory is remembering how to sing a familiar song, such as "Happy Birthday." Procedural memory is a type of nondeclarative memory and involves memory for motor and cognitive skills. Examples of procedural memory include remembering how to tie a shoelace and how to ride a bicycle. Unlike declarative memory, nondeclarative memory remains unchanged across the life span.[4] **Table 1** summarizes the effect of aging on several examples of different types of memory.

Memory can also be broken down into different stages. Acquisition is the ability to encode new information into memory. The rate of acquisition declines across the life span.[21,26] However, retention of information that is successfully learned is preserved in cognitively healthy older adults.[27] Declines also occur in memory retrieval, which is the ability to access newly learned information.[23,26,28]

Language

Language is a complex cognitive domain composed of both crystallized and fluid cognitive abilities. Overall language ability remains intact with aging. Vocabulary

Table 1
Memory and aging

Declines with Age	Remains Stable with Age
Delayed free recall: spontaneous retrieval of information from memory without a cue[23,24] Example: Recalling a list of items to purchase at the grocery store without a cue	Recognition memory: ability to retrieve information when given a cue Example: Correctly giving the details of a story when given yes/no questions
Source memory: knowing the source of the learned information Example: Remembering if you learned a fact because you saw it on television, read it in the newspaper, or heard it from a friend	Temporal order memory: memory for the correct time or sequence of past events Example: Remembering that last Saturday you went to the grocery store after you ate lunch with your friends
Prospective memory: remembering to perform intended actions in the future[25] Example: Remembering to take medicine before going to bed	Procedural memory: memory of how to do things Example: Remembering how to ride a bike

Table 2
Summary of neurocognitive changes with age

	Crystallized vs Fluid	Declines with Age?
Processing speed	Fluid	Yes
Attention	Fluid	Simple tasks: no Complex tasks: yes
Memory	Fluid	Mixed
Language	Crystallized > Fluid	In general: no Visual confrontation naming, verbal fluency: yes
Visuospatial	Mixed	Simple tasks: no Complex tasks: yes
Executive function	Fluid	Mixed

remains stable and even improves over time.[29–32] A few exceptions to the general trend of stability with age are worth mentioning. Visual confrontation naming, or the ability to see a common object and name it, remains about the same until age 70, and then declines in subsequent years.[33] Verbal fluency, which is the ability to perform a word search and generate words for a certain category (eg, letters, animal names) in a certain amount of time, also shows decline with aging.[12,31]

Visuospatial Abilities/Construction

This group of cognitive functions involves the ability to understand space in two and three dimensions. Visual construction skills, which involve the ability to put together individual parts to make a coherent whole (for example, assembling furniture from a box of parts), declines over time.[34] By contrast, visuospatial abilities remain intact. These abilities include object perception (the ability to recognize familiar objects such as household items or faces) and spatial perception (the ability to appreciate the physical location of objects either alone or in relation to other objects).

Executive Functioning

Executive functioning refers to capacities that allow a person to successfully engage in independent, appropriate, purposive, and self-serving behavior. This functioning includes a wide range of cognitive abilities such as the ability to self-monitor, plan, organize, reason, be mentally flexible, and solve problems.[4] Research has shown that concept formation, abstraction, and mental flexibility decline with age, especially after age 70 years,[4] as older adults tend to think more concretely than younger adults.[12,31,35,36] Aging also negatively affects response inhibition, which is the ability to inhibit an automatic response in favor of producing a novel response.[37] Executive abilities requiring a speeded motor component are particularly susceptible to age effects.[30] The Whitehall II study also found declines in inductive reasoning, as measured by verbal and mathematical reasoning tasks, beginning around age 45 years.[31] Reasoning with unfamiliar material also declines with age. Other types of executive function, such as the ability to appreciate similarities, describe the meaning of proverbs, and reason about familiar material, remain stable throughout life.

Summary

Table 2 summarizes key neurocognitive changes seen in normal aging.

STRUCTURAL AND FUNCTIONAL BRAIN CHANGES WITH AGING

Promising developments in neuroscience research may help to explain observed age-related cognitive changes. Studies vary significantly in design, including study population and variables examined, and more research in this area is needed. This section describes some of the age-related changes that have been identified, and presents theories for how these changes may relate to neurocognitive aging.

Decline in Gray Matter Volume

Gray matter volume begins to decrease after age 20 years.[38] The amount of atrophy is most prominent in the prefrontal cortex (**Fig. 1**).

Age-related changes in the temporal lobes are more moderate and involve decreases in the volume of the hippocampus.[39] The entorhinal cortex, which serves as a relay center between the hippocampus and association areas, has been reported to undergo early decreases in volume in Alzheimer dementia (AD), but not in normal aging (**Fig. 2**).[40]

Loss of neurons

The death of neurons themselves has been implicated as a possible cause of loss of gray matter volume. Neuronal death is particularly detrimental, given infrequent cell division and the opportunity for mutations to therefore accumulate.[41]

β-amyloid and its contribution to loss of gray matter volume in normal aging

The protein β-amyloid is found to accumulate in the brains of all patients with AD, and has been proposed to cause AD via neuronal death. Its elevated presence in patients

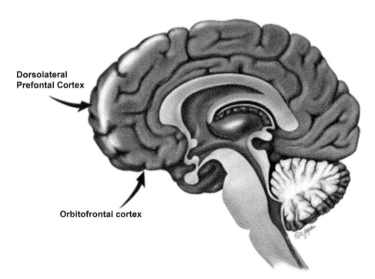

Fig. 1. Prefrontal cortex (orbitofrontal, dorsolateral frontal, and frontopolar regions). Atrophy in this region is associated with deficits in executive function, working memory, and increased perseveration. (*Data from* Raz N, Gunning-Dixon FM, Head D, et al. Neuroanatomical correlates of cognitive aging: evidence from structural magnetic resonance imaging. Neuropsychology 1998;12:95–114; and *Modified from* Dickson VV, Tkacs N, Riegel B. Cognitive influences on self-care decision making in persons with heart failure. Am Heart J 2007;154:424–31.)

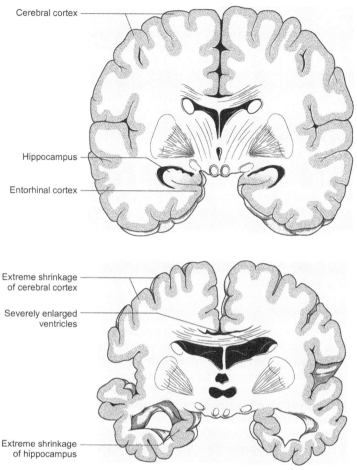

Fig. 2. Hippocampus and entorhinal cortex in normal aging (*above*) and AD (*below*). Atrophy in these regions has been associated with deficits in episodic memory. (*Data from* Raz N, Rodrigue KM, Head D, et al. Differential aging of the medial temporal lobe: a study of a five-year change. Neurology 2004;62:433–8.)

with mild cognitive impairment predicts conversion to AD. In recent years, radiotracers that identify β-amyloid plaques using positron emission tomography (PET) scanners have allowed study of the protein's presence in cognitively intact elderly individuals. β-amyloid is found in the cortex of up to 20% to 30% of normal adults.[42,43] It has been postulated that the presence of β-amyloid in cognitively normal individuals indicates those individuals who eventually will develop AD.[44] One study showed an association between high levels of β-amyloid and both decreased hippocampal volumes and episodic memory in cognitively normal individuals.[45] This finding suggests that amyloid may be an early insult and that it is the downstream effects of its presence, namely cortical volume loss, that lead to clinical change, but this study requires replication with larger sample sizes. Thus, β-amyloid can accumulate in the brains of people currently classified as cognitively normal, but may signal high risk for the development of cognitive impairment over time.

> ### Mentalizing
>
> Mentalizing has been defined as the ability to infer the mental state of others. A recent study using functional magnetic resonance imaging (fMRI) confirmed prior studies showing that older adults have decreased mentalizing capacity.[46] In addition, this decline was also associated with decreases in BOLD (blood-oxygen level dependent) response, a marker for metabolic activity, in the dorsomedial prefrontal cortex. This finding raises the possibility that this area of the brain may be important for mentalizing, and may become less active with advancing age.

Neuronal size and synaptic density

Despite the numerous theories explaining neuronal loss, decline in gray matter volume in older adults is best explained not by death of the neurons themselves but by a decrease in their size and the number of connections between them.[38,47] This reduction in synaptic density is well documented in older adults, and according to the model created by Terry and Katzman,[38] by the age of 130 years a cognitively normal adult will have a synaptic density equivalent to someone with AD. Neurons undergo morphologic changes with aging, including a decrease in the complexity of dendrite arborization, decreased dendrite length, and decreased neuritic spines (the major sites for excitatory synapses). These morphologic changes likely contribute directly to the reduction of synaptic density.[48]

Changes in White Matter

Decreases in white matter volume are much greater than those in gray matter with increasing age.[49] This loss of white matter has been studied with imaging techniques many times, but these investigations have been limited by low numbers of "normal" controls.[50] In one study using morphometric methods from autopsy data of neurologically normal subjects, there was a 16% to 20% decrease in white matter volume in subjects older than 70 years in comparison with younger subjects. This shrinkage of white matter was noted in the precentral gyrus, gyrus rectus, and corpus callosum, areas that demonstrated less than 6% declines in gray matter volume.[51] This study was limited by the small sample size. Nonetheless, these findings have been supported by others; for example, Rogalski and colleagues[52] described that parahippocampal white matter was decreased, leading to decreased communication with hippocampal structures and suggesting a possible mechanism for age-associated decline in memory.

In addition to changes in structure of white matter, a decline in the function of white matter has been studied using diffusion tensor imaging (DTI). DTI has allowed the observation in vivo that white matter integrity declines with increasing age. O'Sullivan and colleagues[53] showed age-related declines in white matter tract integrity are most marked in the anterior white matter and are associated with deficits in executive function. Madden and colleagues[54] showed that loss of integrity of the central portion of the corpus callosum may mediate age-related cognitive decline.

PRACTICAL IMPLICATIONS OF AGE-RELATED COGNITIVE DECLINE

By definition, normal age-related cognitive change does not impair a person's ability to perform daily activities. If an older adult develops functional impairments, it is prudent to pursue a workup for dementia if there is no other obvious explanation for these difficulties, such as a reaction to a medication, a new medical illness, or a vision problem. However, studies show that normal cognitive aging can result in subtle declines in complex functional abilities, such as the ability to drive.[55]

Driving

Data demonstrate that older adults are at higher risk for motor vehicle accidents than are younger drivers.[56] In many cases this is due to mild cognitive impairment (MCI) or dementia, other neurologic or musculoskeletal disorders, medical illness, vision problems, or medications. Unfortunately, even older adults who manage to avoid all of these challenges may still become unsafe drivers because of normal cognitive aging, which can cause small decrements in the multiple cognitive domains needed for driving. These domains include visual attention and processing (the ability to select visual stimuli based on spatial location), visual perception (the ability to accurately perceive and interpret what is seen), executive function, and memory.[57] It is noteworthy that tests of visual processing speed, such as the Useful Field of View test, can predict at-fault motor vehicle crashes in older adults.[58–60]

Despite these observations, many older adults with normal cognition do not experience a decline in driving ability or are able to effectively limit their driving to avoid high-risk situations.[61] The challenge for clinicians is to determine who is able to drive safely, because it has been demonstrated that many older drivers are not able to accurately judge their own driving ability.[62] Unfortunately, many clinicians lack confidence in their ability to assess fitness to drive, and not all clinicians accept that it is their responsibility to do so.[63] Experts recommend that the best way to predict driving fitness is a performance-based road test.[64] This test can be performed by the local Department of Motor Vehicles or by a driver rehabilitation specialist, who is usually an occupational therapist with specialized training in driving skills.

In addition to clinical evaluations, some states use licensure renewal laws as an additional safety net to aid in detecting unsafe older drivers. These laws vary widely from state to state, but in 28 states there are additional requirements that apply only to older drivers, in an effort to identify unsafe drivers.[65] Older driver retraining may be an effective option for older adults who are known to have impaired driving.[66] Older adults suffering only from normal cognitive aging (as opposed to dementia or MCI) seem the most likely to benefit.

Professions with mandatory retirement

Although it is generally illegal in the United States for employers to discriminate against people based on age, there are certain professions, including pilots, air traffic controllers, and federal law enforcement officers, where enforcement of a mandatory retirement age is allowed.[67] The justification for this is that cognitive changes associated with normal cognitive aging, in particular slowing of processing speed, may make it impossible for these professionals to perform their job safely.[68] Unfortunately, these policies are controversial because they fail to take into account individual variability and often are based on limited scientific data.[69,70]

AVOIDING COGNITIVE DECLINE: "SUCCESSFUL" COGNITIVE AGING

There is significant variability in age-related cognitive changes from individual to individual, some of which can be attributed to genetic differences; in fact studies estimate that 60% of general cognitive ability can be attributed to genetics.[71] Medical illness, psychological factors, and sensory deficits such as vision and hearing impairment certainly can also accelerate age-related cognitive decline. The natural question that follows, of course, is whether there are certain environmental factors that can prevent or delay age-associated cognitive declines.

Lifestyle-Cognition Hypothesis

The lifestyle-cognition hypothesis holds that maintaining an active lifestyle and engaging in certain activities during one's life may help prevent age-associated cognitive decline and dementia. Support for this hypothesis is based on the fact that older adults with high cognitive function seem to participate in certain activities with greater frequency than older adults with low cognitive function.[72,73]

Several longitudinal studies, including the Seattle Longitudinal Study, the Bronx Aging Study, and the Victoria Longitudinal Study, have attempted to answer the question of whether certain activities may delay or prevent cognitive decline.[74–76] Many of these studies use performance on cognitive testing as the primary outcome, but more recently investigators have also been using brain structure, for example hippocampal volumes, gray matter atrophy, and white matter lesion load, as outcome measures.[77,78] The box below outlines some of the activities that have been associated with these markers of successful "brain aging."

Activities associated with high cognitive function in older adults

Intellectually Engaging Activities

- Puzzles, discussion groups, reading, using the computer, playing bridge, playing board games, playing musical instruments[75,79–81]
- Careers that involve high complexity[82–84]
- High educational attainment[83,85]

Physical Activities

- Exercise, especially that which improves cardiovascular health[78]
- Gardening[86]
- Dancing[75]

Social engagement

- Travel, cultural events[79,81]
- Socializing with friends and family[79,80]

Studies of lifestyle factors are limited for several reasons. First, they are often based on observational studies, so there is the potential that known or yet unidentified confounders may bias the data. Second, in the case of activities, there is the "which came first, the chicken or the egg" problem with many studies of this type: did a person engage in a particular activity that *prevented* them from developing cognitive decline, or was the person able to engage in that activity *because* they did not experience cognitive decline?[76] There is now a general consensus that AD pathology likely starts decades before symptoms are recognized,[87] so it is entirely possible that study subjects considered cognitively normal could actually be in the preclinical stages of dementia. Third, studies lack consistency and detail in their description and categorization of lifestyle activities, as well as consistency and breadth in the cognitive outcomes measured.[76] More, better, and longer-term longitudinal studies are needed.

Cognitive Reserve

One theory for how certain activities may prevent age-associated cognitive decline is the theory of cognitive reserve. The cognitive reserve hypothesis posits that some individuals have a greater ability to withstand pathologic changes to the brain, such as accumulation of amyloid protein resulting from greater brain reserve.[88] This hypothesis holds that higher levels of education, participation in certain activities, higher socioeconomic status, and baseline intelligence protect against the clinical manifestations of brain disease.[88-90] Passive reserve refers to genetically determined characteristics such as brain volume and the number of neurons and synapses present. Active reserve refers to the brain's potential for plasticity and reorganization in neural processing, allowing it to compensate for neuropathologic changes. The scaffolding theory of aging and cognition (STAC) proposes that alternative neural circuits are recruited to achieve a cognitive goal.[29] The STAC has been supported by several studies regarding the dedifferentiation theory of neurocognitive aging.[91] In these fMRI studies, aging was correlated with recruitment of more areas within a neural network used to perform tasks, especially of working memory and episodic memory, compared with younger controls.[92,93]

Cognitive Retraining

Researchers have demonstrated that subjects can be trained to do better on cognitive testing, and that these improvements can be maintained for years.[74,94] Even more impressive, in the ACTIVE trial, a randomized, multicenter trial involving cognitively normal older adults, cognitive training resulted in less decline in the self-reported ability to perform instrumental activities of daily living after 5 years, in comparison with controls.[94] Cognitive training in this study consisted of 10 1-hour sessions teaching subjects strategies to improve memory, reasoning, and speed of processing. A meta-analysis of speed-of-processing training studies supports the idea that cognitive training can have real effects on cognitively normal subjects' ability to perform activities of daily living.[95] These promising findings suggest that it may be possible to use cognitive training in the future to allow people to minimize functional decline with advancing age. Cognitive training via home videotape has been shown to be 74% as effective as laboratory-based training, offering great potential for making this intervention widely accessible.[96]

SUMMARY

The normal aging process is associated with declines in certain cognitive abilities, such as processing speed and some aspects of memory, language, visuospatial function, and executive function. Although these declines are not yet well understood, promising developments in neurology research have identified declines in volume of gray and white matter as well as changes in white matter function that may contribute to observed cognitive changes with aging. These changes are small and should not result in impairment of function; nonetheless, driving and certain other activities may be compromised, and it is important to detect safety issues early. Participation in certain activities, building cognitive reserve, and engaging in cognitive retraining may all be approaches to achieving successful cognitive aging. Although research in the area of normal cognitive aging may seem less pressing than research in the area of pathologic brain disease, a more complete understanding of normal brain aging may shed light on abnormal brain processes. In addition, the majority of adults older than 65 years will develop neither dementia nor MCI, and more work is needed to better understand how the cognitive function and quality of life of these individuals can be maximized.

REFERENCES

1. Vincent GK, Velkoff VA. The next four decades, the older population in the United States: 2010 to 2050. Washington, DC: U.S. Census Bureau; 2010.

2. Minder CE, Muller T, Gillmann G, et al. Subgroups of refusers in a disability prevention trial in older adults: baseline and follow-up analysis. Am J Public Health 2002;92:445–50.

3. Ford JG, Howerton MW, Lai GY, et al. Barriers to recruiting underrepresented populations to cancer clinical trials: a systematic review. Cancer 2008;112: 228–42.

4. Lezak M, Howieson D, Bigler E, et al. Neuropsychological assessment. 5th edition. New York: Oxford University Press; 2012.

5. Williams JD, Klug MG. Aging and cognition: methodological differences in outcome. Exp Aging Res 1996;22:219–44.

6. Hedden T, Gabrieli JD. Insights into the ageing mind: a view from cognitive neuroscience. Nat Rev Neurosci 2004;5:87–96.

7. Van Beijsterveldt CE, van Boxtel MP, Bosma H, et al. Predictors of attrition in a longitudinal cognitive aging study: the Maastricht Aging Study (MAAS). J Clin Epidemiol 2002;55:216–23.

8. Abner EL, Dennis BC, Mathews MJ, et al. Practice effects in a longitudinal, multicenter Alzheimer's disease prevention clinical trial. Trials 2012;13:217.

9. Salthouse TA. Influence of age on practice effects in longitudinal neurocognitive change. Neuropsychology 2010;24:563–72.

10. Ross GW, Abbott RD, Petrovitch H, et al. Frequency and characteristics of silent dementia among elderly Japanese-American men. The Honolulu-Asia Aging Study. JAMA 1997;277:800–5.

11. Wisdom NM, Mignogna J, Collins RL. Variability in Wechsler Adult Intelligence Scale-IV subtest performance across age. Arch Clin Neuropsychol 2012;27: 389–97.

12. Salthouse TA. Selective review of cognitive aging. J Int Neuropsychol Soc 2010; 16:754–60.

13. Salthouse T. Consequences of age-related cognitive declines. Annu Rev Psychol 2012;63:201–26.

14. Elias L, Saucier D. Neuropsychology: clinical and experimental foundations. Boston: Pearson Education, Inc; 2006.

15. Salthouse TA, Fristoe NM, Lineweaver TT, et al. Aging of attention: does the ability to divide decline? Mem Cognit 1995;23:59–71.

16. Carlson MC, Hasher L, Zacks RT, et al. Aging, distraction, and the benefits of predictable location. Psychol Aging 1995;10:427–36.

17. Salthouse TA, Mitchell DR, Skovronek E, et al. Effects of adult age and working memory on reasoning and spatial abilities. J Exp Psychol Learn Mem Cogn 1989;15:507–16.

18. Luszcz MA, Bryan J. Toward understanding age-related memory loss in late adulthood. Gerontology 1999;45:2–9.

19. Darowski ES, Helder E, Zacks RT, et al. Age-related differences in cognition: the role of distraction control. Neuropsychology 2008;22:638–44.

20. Davis HP, Klebe KJ, Guinther PM, et al. Subjective organization, verbal learning, and forgetting across the life span: from 5 to 89. Exp Aging Res 2013;39:1–26.

21. Delis D, Kramer J, Kaplan E, et al. CVLT-II California verbal learning test. San Antonio (TX): The Psychological Corporation; 2000.

22. Ronnlund M, Nyberg L, Backman L, et al. Stability, growth, and decline in adult life span development of declarative memory: cross-sectional and longitudinal data from a population-based study. Psychol Aging 2005;20:3–18.

23. Price L, Said K, Haaland KY. Age-associated memory impairment of logical memory and visual reproduction. J Clin Exp Neuropsychol 2004;26:531–8.

24. Cargin JW, Maruff P, Collie A, et al. Decline in verbal memory in non-demented older adults. J Clin Exp Neuropsychol 2007;29:706–18.

25. Schnitzspahn KM, Stahl C, Zeintl M, et al. The role of shifting, updating, and inhibition in prospective memory performance in young and older adults. Dev Psychol 2013;49:1544–53.

26. Haaland KY, Price L, Larue A. What does the WMS-III tell us about memory changes with normal aging? J Int Neuropsychol Soc 2003;9:89–96.

27. Whiting WL, Smith AD. Differential age-related processing limitations in recall and recognition tasks. Psychol Aging 1997;12:216–24.

28. Economou A. Memory score discrepancies by healthy middle-aged and older individuals: the contributions of age and education. J Int Neuropsychol Soc 2009;15:963–72.

29. Park DC, Reuter-Lorenz P. The adaptive brain: aging and neurocognitive scaffolding. Annu Rev Psychol 2009;60:173–96.

30. Hayden KM, Welsh-Bohmer KA. Epidemiology of cognitive aging and Alzheimer's disease: contributions of the Cache County Utah study of memory, health and aging. Curr Top Behav Neurosci 2012;10:3–31.

31. Singh-Manoux A, Kivimaki M, Glymour MM, et al. Timing of onset of cognitive decline: results from Whitehall II prospective cohort study. BMJ 2012;344: d7622.

32. Salthouse TA. Decomposing age correlations on neuropsychological and cognitive variables. J Int Neuropsychol Soc 2009;15:650–61.

33. Zec RF, Markwell SJ, Burkett NR, et al. A longitudinal study of confrontation naming in the "normal" elderly. J Int Neuropsychol Soc 2005;11:716–26.

34. Howieson DB, Holm LA, Kaye JA, et al. Neurologic function in the optimally healthy oldest old. Neuropsychological evaluation. Neurology 1993;43: 1882–6.

35. Oosterman JM, Vogels RL, van Harten B, et al. Assessing mental flexibility: neuroanatomical and neuropsychological correlates of the trail making test in elderly people. Clin Neuropsychol 2010;24:203–19.

36. Wecker NS, Kramer JH, Hallam BJ, et al. Mental flexibility: age effects on switching. Neuropsychology 2005;19:345–52.

37. Wecker NS, Kramer JH, Wisniewski A, et al. Age effects on executive ability. Neuropsychology 2000;14:409–14.

38. Terry RD, Katzman R. Life span and synapses: will there be a primary senile dementia? Neurobiol Aging 2001;22:347–8.

39. Raz N, Rodrigue KM, Head D, et al. Differential aging of the medial temporal lobe: a study of a five-year change. Neurology 2004;62:433–8.

40. Braak H, Braak E. Evolution of the neuropathology of Alzheimer's disease. Acta Neurol Scand Suppl 1996;165:3–12.

41. Uttara B, Singh AV, Zamboni P, et al. Oxidative stress and neurodegenerative diseases: a review of upstream and downstream antioxidant therapeutic options. Curr Neuropharmacol 2009;7:65–74.

42. Rodrigue KM, Kennedy KM, Park DC. Beta-amyloid deposition and the aging brain. Neuropsychol Rev 2009;19:436–50.

43. Dickson DW, Crystal HA, Mattiace LA, et al. Identification of normal and pathological aging in prospectively studied nondemented elderly humans. Neurobiol Aging 1992;13:179–89.

44. Pike KE, Savage G, Villemagne VL, et al. Beta-amyloid imaging and memory in nondemented individuals: evidence for preclinical Alzheimer's disease. Brain 2007;130:2837–44.

45. Jack CR Jr, Lowe VJ, Senjem ML, et al. [11]C PiB and structural MRI provide complementary information in imaging of Alzheimer's disease and amnestic mild cognitive impairment. Brain 2008;131:665–80.

46. Moran JM, Jolly E, Mitchell JP. Social-cognitive deficits in normal aging. J Neurosci 2012;32:5553–61.

47. Resnick SM, Pham DL, Kraut MA, et al. Longitudinal magnetic resonance imaging studies of older adults: a shrinking brain. J Neuroscience 2003;23:3295–301.

48. Dickstein DL, Kabaso D, Rocher AB, et al. Changes in the structural complexity of the aged brain. Aging Cell 2007;6:275–84.

49. Salat DH, Kaye JA, Janowsky JS. Prefrontal gray and white matter volumes in healthy aging and Alzheimer disease. Arch Neurol 1999;56:338–44.

50. Sullivan P, Pary R, Telang F, et al. Risk factors for white matter changes detected by magnetic resonance imaging in the elderly. Stroke 1990;21:1424–8.

51. Meier-Ruge W, Ulrich J, Bruhlmann M, et al. Age-related white matter atrophy in the human brain. Ann N Y Acad Sci 1992;673:260–9.

52. Rogalski E, Stebbins GT, Barnes CA, et al. Age-related changes in parahippocampal white matter integrity: a diffusion tensor imaging study. Neuropsychologia 2012;50:1759–65.

53. O'Sullivan M, Summers PE, Jones DK, et al. Normal-appearing white matter in ischemic leukoaraiosis: a diffusion tensor MRI study. Neurology 2001;57:2307–10.

54. Madden DJ, Spaniol J, Costello MC, et al. Cerebral white matter integrity mediates adult age differences in cognitive performance. J Cogn Neurosci 2009;21:289–302.

55. Anstey KJ, Wood J. Chronological age and age-related cognitive deficits are associated with an increase in multiple types of driving errors in late life. Neuropsychology 2011;25:613–21.

56. Braver ER, Trempel RE. Are older drivers actually at higher risk of involvement in collisions resulting in deaths or non-fatal injuries among their passengers and other road users? Inj Prev 2004;10:27–32.

57. Wagner JT, Muri RM, Nef T, et al. Cognition and driving in older persons. Swiss Med Wkly 2011;140:w13136.

58. Owsley C, Ball K, McGwin G Jr, et al. Visual processing impairment and risk of motor vehicle crash among older adults. JAMA 1998;279:1083–8.

59. Friedman C, McGwin G Jr, Ball KK, et al. Association between higher order visual processing abilities and a history of motor vehicle collision involvement by drivers ages 70 and over. Invest Ophthalmol Vis Sci 2013;54:778–82.

60. Ball K, Owsley C. The useful field of view test: a new technique for evaluating age-related declines in visual function. J Am Optom Assoc 1993;64:71–9.

61. Okonkwo OC, Crowe M, Wadley VG, et al. Visual attention and self-regulation of driving among older adults. Int Psychogeriatr 2008;20:162–73.

62. Horswill MS, Sullivan K, Lurie-Beck JK, et al. How realistic are older drivers' ratings of their driving ability? Accid Anal Prev 2013;50:130–7.

63. Marshall S, Demmings EM, Woolnough A, et al. Determining fitness to drive in older persons: a survey of medical and surgical specialists. Can Geriatr J 2012;15:101–19.

64. Carr DB, Ott BR. The older adult driver with cognitive impairment: "It's a very frustrating life". JAMA 2010;303:1632–41.

65. Insurance Institute for Highway Safety. Older drivers: licensing renewal provisions. 2012. Available at: http://www.iihs.org/iihs/topics/laws/olderdrivers?topicName=older-drivers. Accessed September 11, 2013.

66. Korner-Bitensky N, Kua A, von Zweck C, et al. Older driver retraining: an updated systematic review of evidence of effectiveness. J Safety Res 2009;40: 105–11.

67. Payette M, Chatterjee A, Weeks WB. Cost and workforce implications of subjecting all physicians to aviation industry work-hour restrictions. Am J Surg 2009; 197:820–5.

68. Cornell A, Baker SP, Li G. Age-60 Rule: the end is in sight. Aviat Space Environ Med 2007;78:624–6.

69. Taylor JL, Kennedy Q, Noda A, et al. Pilot age and expertise predict flight simulator performance: a 3-year longitudinal study. Neurology 2007;68:648–54.

70. Brand M. Mandatory retirement age debate rages on. National Public Radio 2007. Transcript of a radio show on NPR-hosted by Brand M. Aired August 22, 2007. Available at: http://www.npr.org/templates/story/story.php?storyId=13863666. Accessed September 11, 2013.

71. McClearn GE, Johansson B, Berg S, et al. Substantial genetic influence on cognitive abilities in twins 80 or more years old. Science 1997;276:1560–3.

72. Fratiglioni L, Paillard-Borg S, Winblad B. An active and socially integrated lifestyle in late life might protect against dementia. Lancet Neurol 2004;3:343–53.

73. Marioni RE, van den Hout A, Valenzuela MJ, et al. Active cognitive lifestyle associates with cognitive recovery and a reduced risk of cognitive decline. J Alzheimers Dis 2012;28:223–30.

74. Schaie KW, Willis SL, O'Hanlon AM. Perceived intellectual performance change over seven years. J Gerontol 1994;49:P108–18.

75. Verghese J, Lipton RB, Katz MJ, et al. Leisure activities and the risk of dementia in the elderly. N Engl J Med 2003;348:2508–16.

76. Small BJ, Dixon RA, McArdle JJ, et al. Do changes in lifestyle engagement moderate cognitive decline in normal aging? Evidence from the Victoria Longitudinal Study. Neuropsychology 2012;26:144–55.

77. Fotuhi M, Do D, Jack C. Modifiable factors that alter the size of the hippocampus with ageing. Nat Rev Neurol 2012;8:189–202.

78. Gow AJ, Bastin ME, Munoz Maniega S, et al. Neuroprotective lifestyles and the aging brain: activity, atrophy, and white matter integrity. Neurology 2012;79:1802–8.

79. Crowe M, Andel R, Pedersen NL, et al. Does participation in leisure activities lead to reduced risk of Alzheimer's disease? A prospective study of Swedish twins. J Gerontol B Psychol Sci Soc Sci 2003;58:P249–55.

80. Scarmeas N, Levy G, Tang MX, et al. Influence of leisure activity on the incidence of Alzheimer's disease. Neurology 2001;57:2236–42.

81. Wang HX, Karp A, Winblad B, et al. Late-life engagement in social and leisure activities is associated with a decreased risk of dementia: a longitudinal study from the Kungsholmen project. Am J Epidemiol 2002;155:1081–7.

82. Stern Y, Gurland B, Tatemichi TK, et al. Influence of education and occupation on the incidence of Alzheimer's disease. JAMA 1994;271:1004–10.

83. White L, Katzman R, Losonczy K, et al. Association of education with incidence of cognitive impairment in three established populations for epidemiologic studies of the elderly. J Clin Epidemiol 1994;47:363–74.

84. Woollett K, Maguire EA. Acquiring "the Knowledge" of London's layout drives structural brain changes. Curr Biol 2011;21:2109–14.

85. Wilson RS, Hebert LE, Scherr PA, et al. Educational attainment and cognitive decline in old age. Neurology 2009;72:460–5.

86. Fabrigoule C, Letenneur L, Dartigues JF, et al. Social and leisure activities and risk of dementia: a prospective longitudinal study. J Am Geriatr Soc 1995;43:485–90.

87. Sperling RA, Aisen PS, Beckett LA, et al. Toward defining the preclinical stages of Alzheimer's disease: recommendations from the National Institute on Aging-Alzheimer's Association workgroups on diagnostic guidelines for Alzheimer's disease. Alzheimers Dement 2011;7:280–92.

88. Stern Y. What is cognitive reserve? Theory and research application of the reserve concept. J Int Neuropsychol Soc 2002;8:448–60.

89. Fotenos AF, Mintun MA, Snyder AZ, et al. Brain volume decline in aging: evidence for a relation between socioeconomic status, preclinical Alzheimer disease, and reserve. Arch Neurol 2008;65:113–20.

90. Scarmeas N, Stern Y. Cognitive reserve and lifestyle. J Clin Exp Neuropsychol 2003;25:625–33.

91. Sambataro F, Safrin M, Lemaitre HS, et al. Normal aging modulates prefronto-parietal networks underlying multiple memory processes. Eur J Neurosci 2012;36:3559–67.

92. Cabeza R, Anderson ND, Locantore JK, et al. Aging gracefully: compensatory brain activity in high-performing older adults. Neuroimage 2002;17:1394–402.

93. Cabeza R. Hemispheric asymmetry reduction in older adults: the HAROLD model. Psychol Aging 2002;17:85–100.

94. Willis SL, Tennstedt SL, Marsiske M, et al. Long-term effects of cognitive training on everyday functional outcomes in older adults. JAMA 2006;296:2805–14.

95. Ball K, Edwards JD, Ross LA. The impact of speed of processing training on cognitive and everyday functions. J Gerontol B Psychol Sci Soc Sci 2007; 62(Spec No 1):19–31.

96. Wadley VG, Benz RL, Ball KK, et al. Development and evaluation of home-based speed-of-processing training for older adults. Arch Phys Med Rehabil 2006;87:757–63.

Classification and Epidemiology of MCI

Rosebud Roberts, MS, MB ChB[a,b,*], David S. Knopman, MD[b]

KEYWORDS

- Classification • Epidemiology • Incidence • Mild cognitive impairment • Prevalence
- Risk factors

KEY POINTS

- The prevalence and incidence of mild cognitive impairment (MCI) is high among elderly persons.
- Persons with MCI have a high risk of progression to dementia.
- Several risk factors for MCI are potentially modifiable and amenable to interventions to reduce risk.
- Persons with MCI have a higher mortality than cognitively normal persons.
- Persons with MCI who revert to normal cognition have an increased risk of developing MCI or dementia at a later date.

INTRODUCTION

Mild cognitive impairment (MCI) is the widely used term that describes an intermediate stage from normal cognitive function to dementia. The concept of MCI is highly significant and important to the field of aging and dementia for several reasons. Subjects with MCI have a high rate of progression to dementia over a relatively short period. Even among subjects who revert to normal cognition, the rate of subsequent MCI or dementia is higher than among those who never develop MCI. Research related to MCI provides insights into disease mechanisms in the predementia stage of disease.

Funding Sources: This study was supported by NIH grants P50 AG016574, U01 AG006786, K01 MH068351, and K01 AG028573. This study was also supported by the Driskill Foundation, the Robert Wood Johnson Foundation, and the Robert H. and Clarice Smith and Abigail van Buren Alzheimer's Disease Research Program, and was made possible by the Rochester Epidemiology Project (R01 AG034676).
Conflict of Interest: None.
[a] Division of Epidemiology, Department of Health Sciences Research, Mayo Clinic, 200 First Street Southwest, Rochester, MN 55905, USA; [b] Department of Neurology, Mayo Clinic, 200 First Street Southwest, Rochester, MN 55905, USA
* Corresponding author. Division of Epidemiology, Department of Health Sciences Research, Mayo Clinic, 200 First Street Southwest, Rochester, MN 55905.
E-mail address: roberts.rosebud@mayo.edu

The increasing use of imaging modalities to detect abnormalities in brain structure using magnetic resonance imaging, in vivo imaging of amyloid accumulation using 11C-Pittsburgh Compound-B positron emission tomography (PiB-PET), plaque density using florbetapir F18, and the ability to detect brain hypometabolism using fluorodeoxyglucose (FDG), has shed light on our understanding of the predictors and prognostic markers for MCI and MCI progression to dementia. Furthermore, studies on cerebrospinal fluid (CSF) and other fluid biomarkers will have long-term implications for early detection and treatment of MCI and dementia. Finally, studies on MCI may contribute to development of biomarkers for early detection of MCI, strategies for prevention, and development of therapeutic and nontherapeutic interventions for MCI and dementia. In this review, we present an overview of the classification of MCI, estimates of MCI incidence and prevalence, risk factors for MCI, and the outcomes following an MCI diagnosis.

CLASSIFICATION
Overview

The definition of MCI identifies a symptomatic predementia stage. The earliest reference to MCI described a stage in the severity of dementia[1]; several alternate criteria, mostly related to typical cognitive aging, are not addressed here, but have been described elsewhere.[2,3] In addition to MCI, 2 other classifications that are briefly noted in this article are cognitive impairment, no dementia (CIND), which captures a broader spectrum of cognitive impairment, and MCI due to Alzheimer disease (AD), which primarily identifies persons with an underlying AD pathology.

MCI

MCI identifies a spectrum of disease that includes impairment in both memory and nonmemory cognitive domains.[4–6] This is in contrast to the earlier criteria for MCI in which memory impairment was a requirement for the diagnosis.[7] The criteria for MCI are as follows: cognitive complaint, decline, or impairment; objective evidence of impairment in cognitive domains; essentially normal functional activities; and not demented (**Box 1**).[4,6] The wide spectrum of cognitive and functional impairment that is captured by the MCI designation has an impact on the heterogeneity of outcomes in MCI.

MCI Subtypes

A clinical presentation with memory impairment is characterized as amnestic MCI (aMCI), whereas the absence of memory impairment with presence of impairment in one or more nonmemory cognitive domains, including executive function/attention, language, and visuospatial skills domains, is characterized as nonamnestic MCI (naMCI). This classification by subtype relates to the underlying etiology and pathology, the clinical presentation, and outcomes (**Table 1**). In addition, MCI may consist of impairment in a single cognitive domain or multiple cognitive domains. The number of affected domains has important implications for understanding the extent of the underlying brain disease or pathology, disease severity, and likelihood of progression to dementia. Multiple-domain MCI denotes a greater extent of disease than single-domain MCI, which in turn has implications for a higher rate of progression from MCI to dementia. Information from both the MCI phenotype (aMCI vs. naMCI) and the number of cognitive domains affected (single vs. multiple) is hypothesized to determine future outcomes. Single-domain or multiple-domain aMCI is hypothesized to progress to AD if there is an underlying degenerative etiology.[6] In contrast, naMCI

Box 1
Criteria for MCI and CIND

MCI

Cognitive complaint or concern, cognitive decline or impairment

Objective evidence of impairment in cognitive domains: memory, executive function/attention, language, or visuospatial skills

Essentially normal functional activities

Absence of dementia

CIND

Participant or informant-reported significant decline in cognition or function

Physician-detected significant impairment in cognition

Cognitive test score (s) at least 1.5 SD below the mean of published norms

No clinically important impairment in activities of daily living assessed by physician/informant

Absence of dementia

Abbreviations: CIND, cognitive impairment, no dementia; MCI, mild cognitive impairment.

---

may progress to non-AD dementias, such as frontotemporal dementia, if a single domain is affected with a degenerative etiology or dementia with Lewy bodies if multiple domains are affected with a degenerative etiology.[6] Although there is inadequate research in this area, it is likely that any MCI subtype could precede vascular dementia.

CIND

The concept of CIND is a broader definition of impairment that encompasses subjects who meet criteria for MCI, as well as others who are cognitively impaired but do not meet all the criteria for MCI.[8–10] The criteria for CIND include participant or

---

Table 1
MCI subtypes by etiology, pathology, presentation, and outcomes

Variable	Amnestic	Nonamnestic
Etiology	Neurodegenerative disease APOE ε4	Vascular damage Cerebrovascular disease
Pathology	Neurodegenerative Amyloid β plaques Neurofibrillary tangles Hippocampal atrophy Reduced brain volume	Cerebrovascular Cortical infarctions Subcortical infarctions White matter hyperintensities
Presentation	Memory impairment present	Impairment in nonmemory domains
Long term outcomes	Alzheimer dementia	Non-Alzheimer dementias: Vascular dementia Lewy body Frontotemporal

Abbreviations: APOE, apolipoprotein E; MCI, mild cognitive impairment.

informant-reported significant decline in cognition or function; physician-detected significant impairment in cognition; cognitive test score(s) at least 1.5 SD below the mean compared with normative data; no clinically important impairment in activities of daily living assessed by physician/informant; and absence of dementia (see **Box 1**).

Subtypes of CIND

Subtypes of CIND are based on presumed etiology; they typically include circumscribed (or medically unexplained) memory impairment, delirium, chronic alcohol and drug use, depression, psychiatric illness, mental retardation, and other cognitive impairment. Other subtypes of CIND include medical illness, stroke, or cerebrovascular disease[9]; as many as 12 categories have been noted.[10] To our knowledge, diagnostic criteria using CIND that link the syndrome to biomarkers have not been developed.

MCI due to AD

The classification of MCI due to AD was developed by the National Institute on Aging and the Alzheimer's Association, primarily for research purposes.[11] The motivation was to link the MCI syndrome to a specific etiology by the use of biomarkers for AD. It is based on the clinical criteria for MCI described previously, in combination with additional information from structural magnetic resonance imaging, PiB-PET, FDG-PET, and CSF biomarkers, and determines the certainty with which a person with MCI has underlying AD pathology. This level of certainty is determined from (1) evidence of amyloid β accumulation in the brain assessed by PET and decreased CSF levels of amyloid β (Aβ42), and (2) evidence of neuronal injury assessed as increased CSF tau (total and phosphorylated), brain hypometabolism assessed from [18]fluorodeoxyglucose PET, and hippocampal atrophy from structural magnetic resonance imaging. The utility of this classification is the potential prognostic value for future dementia outcomes. Subjects with a high likelihood of MCI due to AD have a greater certainty of progression to AD. The clinical utility of this classification system remains to be established.

RISK AND PROTECTIVE FACTORS FOR MCI

Several risk factors have been identified for MCI. These include nonmodifiable risk factors, such as age, sex, and genetic factors, and modifiable risk factors, such as level of education, vascular risk factors, cardiovascular outcomes, neuropsychiatric conditions, and imaging biomarkers (**Box 2**). There is a large body of literature on associations of these risk factors with MCI that cannot be thoroughly vetted in this review. In some reports, cognitive and functional severity ratings are considered to be risk or protective factors for progression to dementia, but because the features underlying these ratings are actually metrics for the severity of cerebral dysfunction, these features should be considered in a separate category from demographic, genetic, and medical risk factors.

PREVALENCE AND INCIDENCE OF MCI
MCI Prevalence

Several different criteria have been described for MCI. Therefore, we limited our review of prevalence studies to those that used the more recently published criteria for MCI[4,5,12]; studies with an adequate sample size ($\geq$300 participants); population-based studies; studies that provided a clear description of participant recruitment, clear description of MCI criteria, and how the criteria were operationalized; and studies that recruited participants at 60 years and older. These inclusion criteria

| Box 2 |
| Risk factors for MCI |

Older age

Apoplipoprotein ε4 allele

Sex: Higher in men,[10,36,41,43,46,47] higher in women,[45] and no sex difference[48]

Low number of years of education

Vascular risk factors: Type 2 diabetes, hypertension, obesity, dyslipidemia, smoking

Cardiovascular disease outcomes: coronary artery disease, atrial fibrillation, congestive heart failure, cerebrovascular disease

Systemic inflammation: C-reactive protein

Neuropsychiatric conditions: depression, anxiety, apathy

Protective factors

Higher education

Cognitively stimulating activities

Physical exercise/activities

Dietary factors: monounsaturated and polyunsaturated fatty acids

Mediterranean diet

allowed us to compare estimates across studies of similar design. We also included a few representative studies that used the earlier criteria for aMCI, published criteria for CIND, purely algorithmic criteria for MCI, and a clinic-based study of MCI. However, we excluded studies that were restricted to a narrow age range or to the oldest old (90 years or older),[13,14] because these studies have limited generalizability, and earlier studies that used definitions of cognitive impairment that are not consistent with the current MCI definition, such as benign senescent forgetfulness,[15] age-associated memory impairment,[16] and age-associated cognitive decline.[17]

Prevalence estimates of MCI ranged from 16% to 20% for most of the reviewed studies (**Table 2**). A few studies had very high estimates that could be due to issues with nonparticipation or elements peculiar to the study.[18] Estimates from studies conducted in urban sites, multiethnic cohorts, and in clinic-based studies were also at the higher end of the spectrum.

MCI Incidence

In contrast to prevalence studies, there are fewer studies on MCI incidence rates.[19] There is a wide range of incidence rates (1000 person years) from 5.1 to 168.0 (**Table 3**). A few studies reported estimates of incident aMCI only; these ranged from 10 to 14. The key risk factors for MCI described from these incident studies included older age, low education, and APOE ε4 allele. In addition, cardiovascular disease (type 2 diabetes), black and Hispanic ethnicity, subjective memory complaints, and stroke have also been associated with incident MCI.

MCI OUTCOMES
Progression to Dementia

An important MCI outcome is the increased risk of progression to dementia.[20] In fact, the designation of MCI, in addition to characterizing a particular level of cognitive and

Table 2
Prevalence rates for MCI

Publication	Country	Design and Criteria for MCI	n	Age (y)	Prevalence (%)
Hanninen et al,[36] 2002	Kuopio, Finland	Population-based sample.	806	60–76	Overall, 6.5%. aMCI, 5.3%. Age 60–64 y, 2.4%; 65–69, 4.8%; 70–76, 8.4% Men, 7.1%; women, 4.1%
Busse et al,[37] 2003	Leipzig Longitudinal Study of the Aged, Germany	Population-based, prospective, community-dwelling cohort.	929	≥75	Overall, 5.1%. Age 75–79 y, 4.7%; 80–84, 5.6%; ≥85, 5.2%.
Fisk et al,[49] 2003	Canadian Study of Health and Aging, Canada	Population-based, aMCI criteria. Urban and rural cohort.	1790	≥65	aMCI, 2.4%. No sex-specific or age-specific estimates provided.
Lopez et al,[48] 2003	Cardiovascular Health Study, US	Representative prospective, multiethnic, cohort. Predominantly urban setting.	2470	≥75	Overall, 18.8%. Age <75 y, 18.8%; 75–79, 14.7%; 80–84, 22.6%; ≥85, 28.9%. Men, 19%; women, 18.7%.
Manly et al,[39] 2005	North Manhattan study, US	Prospective, population-based, multiethnic cohort. MCI criteria. Urban setting.	1315	≥65	Overall, 28.3%. Age 65–75 y, 24.0%; >75, 32.6%. No sex difference.
Busse et al,[50] 2006	Leipzig Longitudinal Study of the Aged, Germany	Population-based, prospective study. Community dwelling cohort.	980	≥75	Overall, 19.4% (9.3% if subjective memory complaint criterion excluded). No age-specific and sex-specific rates reported.
Das et al,[51] 2007	Kolkata, India	Cross-sectional design. Systematic random sampling within city blocks, random sampling within households. Urban setting. aMCI criteria and multiple domain.[a]	745	≥50	aMCI, 14.9%. Age 50–59 y, 12.4%; 60–64, 17.4%; 65–69, 11.7%; 70–74, 12.3%; 75–79, 17.9%; ≥80, 10.6%. Men, 7.6%; women, 4.5%. Multiple domain: men, 6.3%; women, 11.4%.
Artero et al,[40] 2008	3-city study, France	Population-based, community dwelling: Revised published MCI consensus criteria.	6892	≥65	Overall, 42% (frequency).

Study	Study Name	Description	N	Age	Prevalence
Petersen et al,[46] 2010	Mayo Clinic Study of Aging	Population-based, Published MCI criteria.	1969	70–89	Overall, 16.0%. Age 70–79 y, 12.1%; 80–89, 22.2%. Men, 19.0%; women, 14.1%
Sachdev et al,[18] 2012	Sydney Memory and Aging Study, Australia	Population-based. Published MCI criteria.	757	70–90	Overall, 39.1%. Age 70–79 y, 36.7%; 80–89: 43.3%. Men: 70–79, 41.9%; ≥80, 43.6%. Women: 70–79, 32.2%; ≥80, 43.0%.
Unverzagt et al,[9] 2001	Indianapolis Study of Health and Aging, Indianapolis, US	Representative sample of community-dwelling, African American, CIND.	2212	≥65	Overall, 23.4%. Age 65–74 y, 19.2%; 75–84, 27.6%; ≥85, 38%.
Plassman et al,[10] 2008	Aging, Demographics, and Memory Study, US	Population-based, nationally representative criteria: exclusion of dementia and other impairments, cognitive testing battery, CIND.	856	≥71	Overall, 22.2%. Age 71–79 y,16.0%; 80–89, 29.2%; ≥90, 39.0%. Men vs. women: OR, 1.62 (95% CI 1.09–2.41).
Luck et al,[45] 2007	Aging, Cognition, Dementia in Primary Care Patients, Germany	General practice; clinic-based. Published MCI criteria.	3242	≥75	Overall, 25.2%. Age 75–79 y, 24.6%; 80–84, 24.2%; 85–98, 32.8%. Women vs. men; OR, 1.36 (95% CI 1.14–1.63)
Ganguli et al,[43] 2004	Monongahela Valley Independent Elders Survey, US	Representative community-based, prospective cohort, aMCI criteria applied to previously collected data. Algorithmic criteria.[a]	1248	≥75	Overall, 6.3%. No age-specific rates. Men vs. women: OR, 1.9 (95% CI 1.3–2.8; P = .001).
Ganguli et al,[44] 2010	Monongahela-Youghiogheny Healthy Aging Team Project, US	Population-based. Purely cognitively defined MCI, modified expanded MCI criteria; algorithmic classification.[a]	1982	≥65	Overall, 17.8%. Age 65–74 y, 17.5%; 75–84, 18.0%; ≥85, 18.5%.

Abbreviations: aMCI, amnestic MCI; CI, confidence interval; CIND, cognitive impairment, no dementia; MCI, mild cognitive impairment; OR, odds ratio.
[a] Based on neuropsychological testing.

Table 3
Incidence rates and risk factors for MCI

Incidence Studies	Study, Country	Design, Follow-up	n	Age (y)	Incidence (per 1000 Person Years) or Frequency (%)	Risk Factors
Larrieu et al,[52] 2002	Personnes Agees QUID study, France	Population-based, 5 y.	1265	≥65	9.9/1000 (aMCI)	Female sex, higher education.
Busse et al,[37] 2003	Leipzig Longitudinal Study of the Aged, Germany	Population-based, 1756 person years	684	≥75	8.5/1000 (aMCI) 12.2/1000 (any MCI)	Not reported.
Tervo et al,[53] 2004	Kuopio, Finland	Population-based, 3.3 y (aMCI criteria).	550	60–76	25.9/1000 person years (aMCI)	Older age, low education, APOE ε4, treated hypertension, cardiovascular disease.
Solfrizzi et al,[54] 2004	Italian Longitudinal Study on Aging, Italy	Population-based, 3.5 y follow-up (retroactively applied MCI criteria).	2963	65–84	21.5/1000 person years	Older age, low education.
Palmer et al,[55] 2008	Kungsholmen Project, Sweden	Population-based; 3.4 y	379	≥75	168/1000; single-domain aMCI, 34/1000; single-domain naMCI, 82/1000; multiple-domain MCI, 52/1000 person years	Not reported.
Carraciolo et al,[56] 2008	Kungsholmen Project, Sweden	Population-based; 9 y (4292 person years)	1070	≥75	aMCI, 13.7/1000; other cognitive impairment, 42.1/1000.	Older age, higher risk in men.

Source	Study, Location	Design	N	Age	Incidence	Risk Factors
Manly et al,[57] 2008	North Manhattan study, US	Multiracial cohort; mean 4.7 y (7504.9 person years of follow-up)	1800	≥65	Overall, incidence 5.1%. aMCI, 2.3%; naMCI, 2.8/%	Older age; ethnicity, black or Hispanic greater than white ethnicity; hypertension.
Ravaglia et al,[58] 2008	Conselice Study of Brain Aging, Italy	Population-based, mean, 3.8 y	685	≥65	76.8/1000	Not reported.
Luck et al,[59] 2010	Leipzig Longitudinal Study of Aging, Germany	Population-based, 8 y of follow-up.	519	≥75	Overall: 76.5/1000 person years aMCI: 27.9/1000 person years naMCI: 48.6/1000 person years	Older age, subjective memory complaints, impaired functional status.
Roberts et al,[41] 2012	Mayo Clinic Study of Aging, USA	Population-based; 3.4 y follow-up	1450	≥70	63.6 per 1000 person years aMCI; 37.7; naMCI:14.7	Older age, male sex, low education.
Luck et al,[60] 2010	German Study on Aging, Cognition and Dementia in Primary Care Patients, Germany	Community-dwelling patients of general practitioners; 3 y (6198 person years)	2331	≥75	56.5/1000 person years aMCI: 12.3/1000, naMCI: 49.8/1000 Age: 75–79; 52.7; 80–84; 55.4, ≥85, 94.0. Men, 60.4; women, 54.4.	Older age, stroke, APOE ε4 allele, subjective memory complaints.

Abbreviations: aMCI, amnestic MCI; MCI, mild cognitive impairment; naMCI, non-amnestic MCI.

functional impairment, also carries with it a prognosis that is decidedly less favorable than persons with normal cognition. Most studies reported rates of progression from MCI to dementia from 20% to 40% (10%–15% per year) with a few outliers at the lower and higher ends of the spectrum (**Table 4**). Several of the studies also demonstrate that subjects with MCI progress to dementia at a higher rate than cognitively normal subjects. These studies indicate that a higher frequency of subjects with MCI remain in the MCI stage or progress to dementia than revert to normal cognition.

Risk Factors for Progression to Dementia

Interestingly, risk factors for progression have not been consistently found to be the same as the risk factors for incident MCI (see **Table 4**). For example, some studies have observed an association of vascular risk factors with progression to dementia,[21,22] but others have not.[23] However, markers for the severity of the underlying pathology and cerebral dysfunction have more consistently been associated with progression to dementia. These include the degree of functional impairment, severity of neuropsychological test scores,[24] and presence of neuropsychiatric behaviors[25] at the time of MCI diagnosis. In addition, abnormalities in structural magnetic resonance imaging (eg, hippocampal atrophy, volumetric brain changes) and magnetic resonance spectroscopy of the brain are associated with increased risk of progression.[26,27]

MCI Reversion to Normal

An interesting outcome of MCI is that of reversion to normal cognitive function at a subsequent evaluation (see **Table 4**). Rather than representing a flaw in the concept, the observations of reversion to normal among individuals points out an inherent clinical feature of the syndrome, namely that its severity exhibits slow oscillations over time. On average, about 20% of subjects with MCI will improve over time. Despite this, subjects who revert to normal cognition may not be altogether cognitively normal. These subjects have a greater likelihood of progression to MCI or dementia at a subsequent evaluation than do subjects who never developed MCI (Roberts RO, 2013, unpublished data).[28,29] This suggests that subjects who revert to normal may already have some degree of underlying brain pathology.

Risk Factors for Reversion

Risk factors for reversion to normal appear, in general, to be the opposite of those that predict progression to dementia (see **Table 4**). Factors that have been associated with increased risk of reversion to normal include demographic factors: younger age, male sex; markers of MCI severity at the time of diagnosis: single-domain MCI, higher Mini-Mental State Examination (MMSE), lower Clinical Dementia Rating Scale (CDR) sum of boxes, MCI type (naMCI), lower Functional Activities Questionnaire score; absence of medical conditions; and alcohol abuse (reversible condition). One study suggested that reversion to normal was less likely with higher than lower levels of education.[30] This may be consistent with studies that suggest that higher levels of education provide greater cognitive reserve that may reduce the clinical expression of symptoms; however, they may have greater underlying disease pathology at the time of presentation of MCI or dementia.[31–33]

MCI Mortality

There are relatively few studies on mortality in persons with MCI. These studies suggest an increased mortality among subjects with MCI compared with cognitively normal subjects.[10,34,35] In one study, however, the rate (per 1000 person years) was higher in cognitively normal subjects than in MCI cases (27.0) who progressed to dementia (41.3).[29] This may have occurred because the period of follow-up was assessed from the time when participants were cognitively normal rather than when they had MCI or dementia, thus attributing a longer follow-up to MCI cases by including times when subjects did not actually have MCI or dementia.

DISCUSSION

MCI is an important public health concern because of the increased risk of progression to dementia and increased mortality. However, certain issues hinder the clinical utility of the diagnosis. In particular, cognitive and functional severity within the MCI definition varies over a wide range, so that the syndrome of MCI is not homogeneous. The variability in prevalence rates, incidence rates, and rates of progression to dementia underscores the need to recognize that heterogeneity, and to develop standardized criteria for diagnosis of MCI that are easy to operationalize, have high reliability and validity in the clinical setting, and yield consistent estimates across studies. The clinical utility of imaging and CSF biomarkers in the diagnosis of MCI is yet to be established; however, there are strong suggestions from the research literature that including these biomarkers in the MCI criteria may result in a greater sensitivity and specificity of the MCI diagnosis, greater positive and negative predictive value, and may have greater prognostic implications than the current MCI definition. There is considerable research yet to be done before the biomarkers can be used for diagnosis in routine clinical care. Factors that would limit their inclusion in routine care, however, include the cost of the imaging procedures and the invasiveness of the lumbar puncture to acquire CSF.

Variability in Estimates of MCI Prevalence and Incidence

Several methodological reasons have been proposed for varying estimates of MCI prevalence and incidence across studies. These include the source of subjects (population-based vs. clinic-based), the criteria used for MCI, how these MCI criteria were operationalized, domain scores versus single global tests, cut-points for abnormality for neuropsychological test scores (≥ 1.0 SD vs. ≥ 1.5 SD), number of tests used to assess abnormality, and the use of clinical versus algorithmic approaches (not informant based) to assign an MCI diagnosis. Although there were relatively few outliers in the selected studies for prevalence, there were some differences. Studies in Europe, specifically Finland and Germany, reported lower estimates of prevalence[36,37] than the more comparable estimates reported across the US studies.[38] In the United States, estimates were higher for studies in larger cities[39,40] and studies including ethnic groups other than whites.[9] Differences in how MCI criteria were applied may have resulted in higher estimates of prevalence in the Sydney and Aging Study in Australia[18] than in the Mayo Clinic Study of Aging in the United States,[41] even though the study designs were similar. The original description of the MCI criteria was intended to guide clinicians rather than to be used as absolute cut-points for assigning abnormality.[42] Even when an algorithmic classification was used in 2 studies, retrospective application of MCI criteria to previously collected data yielded low estimates of prevalence[43] compared with concurrent application of MCI criteria.[44] As expected, the estimate from a clinic-based design was on the higher end of the spectrum.[45] Finally, estimates across studies may vary when a single test was used to assess cognition, and whether or not cognitive test scores were compared with normative data.

The variability in incidence rates across studies was even greater than for prevalence estimates. This could be due to the same issues as for prevalence (differences in sample size, MCI criteria used and how they were operationalized, cut-points for

Table 4
Rates of progression from MCI to dementia, predictors of progression and reversion from MCI to normal cognition

Citation	Study	MCI Cases, Years of Follow-up	Progression to Dementia (1000 pyrs) or Frequency MCI (% Who Progressed)	Predictors of Progression	Reversion Rate (% Who Reverted to Normal), Predictors
Unverzagt et al,[9] 2001	Indianapolis Study of Health and Aging, Indianapolis, US	Prevalent cases, 66. Follow-up, 18 mo.	26% progressed to dementia; 50% had stable CIND.	Stroke or cerebrovascular disease, medically unexplained memory loss.	24% reversion. Highest rates: other/indeterminate subjects, with alcohol abuse.
Larrieu et al,[52] 2002	Personnes Agées Quid, France	Prevalent or incident MCI, 409 cases. Follow-up, 5 y.	8.3% per y Progression to AD: aMCI: 83/1000 pyrs, OCIND, 71/1000 pyrs. Non-AD dementia: aMCI, 7.5/1000 pyrs OCIND, 17/1000 pyrs.	aMCI predicted AD. OCIND predicted non-AD dementia.	41% reversion in prevalent MCI cases at 2-y follow-up.
Solfrizzi et al,[54] 2004	Italian Longitudinal Study on Aging, Italy	Prevalent MCI, 72 cases with follow-up. Follow-up, 3.5 y.	Progression, 38/1000 pyrs; 20.8% progressed; 41.7% remained MCI or declined further.	Stroke. No age or sex association.	37.5% reversion.
Artero et al,[40] 2008	3 Cities Study, France	Prevalent MCI, 2882 cases. Follow-up, 4 y.	6.6% (n =189) incident dementia, 56.5% stable MCI.	APOE ε4 allele, stroke, low education, impaired IADL, older age, hypertension, diabetes, stroke, subclinical depression, anticholinergic drugs, poor health status.	37% reversion. Men (39%) more likely to revert to normal vs. women (36%, $P = .02$).

Study	Setting	Sample	Progression	Factors	Reversion
Manly et al,[57] 2008	North Manhattan Study, US	Prevalent or incident MCI, 564 cases. Follow-up, 4.7 y.	21.8% MCI progressed to AD (5.4% per y) vs. 10.3% progression in cognitively normal. Stable MCI: 46.5%.	Older age, lower education, ethnicity (black, Hispanic), APOE ε4 allele, type 2 diabetes, stroke, multidomain MCI.	30.2% reversion. Highest reversion rate for single-domain MCI, lowest rate for multiple-domain MCI.
Plassman et al,[10] 2008	Aging, Demographics, and Memory Study, US	Prevalent MCI, n = 180. Mean follow-up, 17 mo.	16.7% progression to dementia (11.7% per y): 63.8% had stable MCI.	Older age, lower education, trend for women. No association with race or APOE ε4 allele.	19.6% reversion.
Ravaglia et al,[58] 2008	Conselice Study of Brain Aging, Italy	Prevalent MCI: n = 60 cases. Follow-up, 3.8 y.	41.7% progressed to dementia (14% per y vs. 4% in cognitively normal). Among 20 MCI cases who were fully evaluated at follow-up and did not have dementia. 65% had stable MCI.	Older age, APOE ε4 allele, women, low level of education, lower MMSE scores, aMCI, multidomain MCI.	35% reversion among 20 MCI cases who were fully evaluated at follow-up and did not have dementia.
Palmer et al,[55] 2008	Kungsholmen Project, Sweden	Prevalent MCI, n = Follow-up, 3.4 y.	20.3% of 350 had incident dementia (77.5% had AD).	Progression higher with multidomain MCI (HR, 23.6) and aMCI (HR, 17.9).	Not reported
Farias et al,[24] 2009	University of California Alzheimer's disease Center, US	Clinic and community-based participants, 111 cases. Follow-up 2.4 y.	Total sample: 10% per y conversion to dementia; 13% for clinic sample: 3% per y for community sample.	Clinic recruitment, CDR at baseline (ie, functional impairment), white matter hyperintensity volume.	Not reported

(continued on next page)

Table 4
(continued)

Citation	Study	MCI Cases, Years of Follow-up	Progression to Dementia (1000 pyrs) or Frequency MCI (% Who Progressed)	Predictors of Progression	Reversion Rate (% Who Reverted to Normal), Predictors
Luck et al,[61] 2012	German study on Aging, Cognition, and Dementia in Primary Care Patients, Germany	Prevalent MCI, 483 cases. Follow-up, 4.5 y.	Progression, 73/1000 pyrs (24.2%) in MCI cases vs. 21.6/1000 pyrs (8.2%) in cognitively normal.	Impairment in IADL, older age, stroke, depressive symptoms, APOE ε4 allele.	Not reported.
Mauri et al,[62] 2012	Laboratory of Neuropsychology & Alzheimer's Assessment Unit, Italy	Clinic-based 208 patients with aMCI. Follow-up, 6 y. Case-control design.	68% progression.	Neuropsychiatric symptoms (Neuropsychiatric Inventory score ≥4); apathy.	Not reported.
Han et al,[30] 2012	Korean Longitudinal Study on Health and Aging, Korea	Prevalent MCI, 140 cases. Mean follow-up, 1.57 y.	13.6% progressed to dementia (8.64% per y conversion); 57.9% had stable MCI.	Multidomain MCI, low MMSE score.	28.6% reversion, (18.2% per y). Lower rate of reversion: multidomain MCI, higher education, higher MMSE score.
Peters et al,[63] 2012	Cache County Study of Memory Health and Aging, US	Prevalent CIND, 230 cases. Follow-up, 3.3 y.	37.0% progressed to dementia (12.2% per y); 63% had stable MCI.	Older age, APOE ε4 allele low MMSE, high CDR Sum of boxes neuropsychiatric symptoms, nighttime behaviors.	

Lopez et al,[29] 2012	Pittsburgh Cardiovascular Health Study, US	Incident MCI, 200 cases. Follow-up, mean, 2.8 y.	53.5% progressed to dementia; 46.5% had stable MCI.	Older age, women, lower MMSE score.	20% reversion.
Koepsell et al,[28] 2012	Participants recruited from 33 Alzheimer's Disease Centers, US	Prevalent and incident MCI: n = 3020. Follow-up: 3 y.	20% progressed to dementia; 64% had stable MCI.	Not reported.	16% reversion over 1 y. Higher risk for younger age, no APOE ε4; higher MMSE, lower CDR sum of boxes, aMCI, multidomain MCI, low FAQ score.
Roberts RO; Neurology 2013 (unpublished data)	Mayo Clinic Study of Aging, US	MCI cases: 534 (282 prevalent, 252 incident). Follow-up, median 2.5 y.	Incidence: 71.3 per 1000 pyrs. 26.0% progressed to dementia; 36.3 had stable MCI.	Higher progression rates for women, aMCI, and multidomain MCI.	37.6% (175 per 1000 pyrs). Lower risk for aMCI, multidomain MCI, APOE ε4 allele, high FAQ score, not married.

Abbreviations: aMCI, amnestic MCI; APOE, apolipoprotein E; CDR, Clinical Dementia Rating Scale; FAQ, Functional Activities Questionnaire; IADL, instrumental activities of daily living; MCI, mild cognitive impairment; MMSE, Mini-Mental State Examination; naMCI, nonamnestic MCI; OCIND, other cognitive impairment, not demented; pyrs, person years.

cognitive scores), but also to differences in duration of follow-up for end points.[38] It is not sufficient to compare summary rates only; comparison of age-specific rates are important because MCI is an age-related condition. However, not all studies provide age-specific rates, and when they do, age ranges for estimates are not consistent across studies.[38] Although most studies reported rates per 1000 person years, some studies only reported the percentage of people who had progressed from MCI to normal, making it even more difficult to compare rates across studies.

Clinical Implications of MCI Progression, Reversion, and Mortality

The high rate of progression to dementia among subjects with MCI emphasizes the need to identify methods to prevent MCI, reduce the burden of MCI, and identify those at increased risk of MCI who may benefit from early interventions. Furthermore, considering that a high proportion of risk factors are preventable, it is essential that physicians and health care personnel (1) educate their patients on how to reduce their risk of MCI through dietary measures, exercise, engagement in cognitively stimulating activities, and stroke prevention; (2) detect and reduce risk factors and achieve adequate control of cardiovascular risk factors and outcomes; and (3) initiate nontherapeutic and therapeutic interventions when they become available. These measures should have the potential to reduce the risk of MCI, with direct beneficial implications for progression from MCI to dementia, and reduced mortality from MCI.

Several studies have now established that subjects with MCI may improve to a cognitively normal state at a subsequent follow-up. This phenomenon has been observed not only in population-based studies with a milder disease spectrum of MCI cases, but also among subjects seen at memory clinics where a narrower and more severe disease spectrum of MCI would be expected.[28] This suggests that the phenomenon is real and not simply a function of diagnostic characterization, but may actually be due to oscillations or variations in manifestation of symptoms from one evaluation to the next, until the all-absorbing state of dementia occurs. Subjects who revert to normal after MCI may differ from subjects who never receive a diagnosis of MCI. The higher risk of progression to MCI or dementia in persons who revert to cognitively normal, suggests the presence of an underlying brain pathology. These subjects require active follow-up and timely intervention to prevent decline to dementia.

SUMMARY

MCI is a stage that is potentially amenable to interventions that may prevent further decline to dementia, the stage of cognitive impairment that has more substantial impact on daily function. The classification of MCI is improving over time, and inclusion of imaging and other biomarkers may further enhance the detection of subjects with MCI. This would facilitate comparisons across studies, contribute to better selection of subjects for clinical trials, enhance the detection of clinical trials outcomes, provide a better understanding of MCI outcomes, and contribute to early detection of subjects with MCI. Subjects with MCI may benefit from interventions that will reduce their risk of progression to dementia, and may be eligible for treatment with disease-modifying drugs that reverse previous damage or prevent further decline, when such treatments become available.

REFERENCES

1. Reisberg B, Ferris S, de Leon M, et al. Stage-specific behavioral, cognitive, and in vivo changes in community residing subjects with age-associated memory

impairment and primary degenerative dementia of the Alzheimer type. Drug Dev Res 1988;15:101–14.

2. Bischkopf J, Busse A, Angermeyer MC. Mild cognitive impairment—a review of prevalence, incidence and outcome according to current approaches. Acta Psychiatr Scand 2002;106:403–14.

3. Stephan BC, Matthews FE, McKeith IG, et al. Early cognitive change in the general population: how do different definitions work? J Am Geriatr Soc 2007;55: 1534–40.

4. Petersen RC. Mild cognitive impairment as a diagnostic entity. J Intern Med 2004;256:183–94.

5. Winblad B, Palmer K, Kivipelto M, et al. Mild cognitive impairment—beyond controversies, towards a consensus: report of the International Working Group on Mild Cognitive Impairment. J Intern Med 2004;256:240–6.

6. Petersen RC, Roberts RO, Knopman DS, et al. Mild cognitive impairment: ten years later. Arch Neurol 2009;66:1447–55.

7. Petersen RC, Smith GE, Waring SC, et al. Mild cognitive impairment: clinical characterization and outcome. Arch Neurol 1999;56:303–8.

8. Graham JE, Rockwood K, Beattie BL, et al. Prevalence and severity of cognitive impairment with and without dementia in an elderly population. Lancet 1997; 349:1793–6.

9. Unverzagt FW, Gao S, Baiyewu O, et al. Prevalence of cognitive impairment: data from the Indianapolis Study of Health and Aging. Neurology 2001;57:1655–62.

10. Plassman BL, Langa KM, Fisher GG, et al. Prevalence of cognitive impairment without dementia in the United States. Ann Intern Med 2008;148:427–34.

11. Albert MS, DeKosky ST, Dickson D, et al. The diagnosis of mild cognitive impairment due to Alzheimer's disease: recommendations from the National Institute on Aging–Alzheimer's Association workgroups on diagnostic guidelines for Alzheimer's disease. Alzheimers Dement 2011;7:270–9.

12. Petersen RC. Does the source of subjects matter? Absolutely! Neurology 2010; 74:1754–5.

13. Jungwirth S, Weissgram S, Zehetmayer S, et al. VITA: subtypes of mild cognitive impairment in a community-based cohort at the age of 75 years. Int J Geriatr Psychiatry 2005;20:452–8.

14. Pioggiosi PP, Berardi D, Ferrari B, et al. Occurrence of cognitive impairment after age 90: MCI and other broadly used concepts. Brain Res Bull 2006;68:227–32.

15. Kral VA. Senescent forgetfulness: benign and malignant. Can Med Assoc J 1962;86:257–60.

16. Crook T, Bartus R, Ferris S, et al. Age associated memory impairment: proposed diagnostic criteria and measures of clinical change: report of a National Institute of Mental Health Work Group. Dev Neuropsychol 1986;2:261–76.

17. Levy R. Aging-associated cognitive decline. Working Party of the International Psychogeriatric Association in collaboration with the World Health Organization. Int Psychogeriatr 1994;6:63–8.

18. Sachdev PS, Lipnicki DM, Crawford J, et al. Risk profiles for mild cognitive impairment vary by age and sex: the Sydney Memory and Ageing Study. Am J Geriatr Psychiatry 2012;20:854–65.

19. Luck T, Luppa M, Briel S, et al. Incidence of mild cognitive impairment: a systematic review. Dement Geriatr Cogn Disord 2010;29:164–75.

20. Mitchell AJ, Shiri-Feshki M. Rate of progression of mild cognitive impairment to dementia—meta-analysis of 41 robust inception cohort studies. Acta Psychiatr Scand 2009;119:252–65.

21. Xu W, Caracciolo B, Wang HX, et al. Accelerated progression from mild cognitive impairment to dementia in people with diabetes. Diabetes 2010;59: 2928–35.
22. Di Carlo A, Lamassa M, Baldereschi M, et al. CIND and MCI in the Italian elderly: frequency, vascular risk factors, progression to dementia. Neurology 2007;68: 1909–16.
23. DeCarli C, Mungas D, Harvey D, et al. Memory impairment, but not cerebrovascular disease, predicts progression of MCI to dementia. Neurology 2004;63: 220–7.
24. Farias ST, Mungas D, Reed BR, et al. Progression of mild cognitive impairment to dementia in clinic- vs community-based cohorts. Arch Neurol 2009;66: 1151–7.
25. Palmer K, Berger AK, Monastero R, et al. Predictors of progression from mild cognitive impairment to Alzheimer disease. Neurology 2007;68:1596–602.
26. Kantarci K, Weigand SD, Przybelski SA, et al. Risk of dementia in MCI: combined effect of cerebrovascular disease, volumetric MRI, and 1H MRS. Neurology 2009;72:1519–25.
27. Amieva H, Letenneur L, Dartigues JF, et al. Annual rate and predictors of conversion to dementia in subjects presenting mild cognitive impairment criteria defined according to a population-based study. Dement Geriatr Cogn Disord 2004;18:87–93.
28. Koepsell TD, Monsell SE. Reversion from mild cognitive impairment to normal or near-normal cognition: risk factors and prognosis. Neurology 2012;79:1591–8.
29. Lopez OL, Becker JT, Chang YF, et al. Incidence of mild cognitive impairment in the Pittsburgh cardiovascular health study-cognition study. Neurology 2012;79: 1599–606.
30. Han JW, Kim TH, Lee SB, et al. Predictive validity and diagnostic stability of mild cognitive impairment subtypes. Alzheimers Dement 2012;8:553–9.
31. Meng X, D'Arcy C. Education and dementia in the context of the cognitive reserve hypothesis: a systematic review with meta-analyses and qualitative analyses. PLoS One 2012;7:e38268.
32. Brayne C, Ince PG, Keage HA, et al. Education, the brain and dementia: neuroprotection or compensation? Brain 2010;133:2210–6.
33. Stern Y. What is cognitive reserve? Theory and research application of the reserve concept. J Int Neuropsychol Soc 2002;8:448–60.
34. Hunderfund AL, Roberts RO, Slusser TC, et al. Mortality in amnestic mild cognitive impairment: a prospective community study. Neurology 2006;67:1764–8.
35. Bennett DA, Wilson RS, Schneider JA, et al. Natural history of mild cognitive impairment in older persons. Neurology 2002;59:198–205.
36. Hanninen T, Hallikainen M, Tuomainen S, et al. Prevalence of mild cognitive impairment: a population-based study in elderly subjects. Acta Neurol Scand 2002;106:148–54.
37. Busse A, Bischkopf J, Riedel-Heller SG, et al. Mild cognitive impairment: prevalence and incidence according to different diagnostic criteria. Results of the Leipzig Longitudinal Study of the Aged (LEILA75+). Br J Psychiatry 2003; 182:449–54.
38. Ward A, Arrighi HM, Michels S, et al. Mild cognitive impairment: disparity of incidence and prevalence estimates. Alzheimers Dement 2012;8:14–21.
39. Manly JJ, Bell-McGinty S, Tang MX, et al. Implementing diagnostic criteria and estimating frequency of mild cognitive impairment in an urban community. Arch Neurol 2005;62:1739–46.

40. Artero S, Ancelin ML, Portet F, et al. Risk profiles for mild cognitive impairment and progression to dementia are gender specific. J Neurol Neurosurg Psychiatry 2008;79:979–84.
41. Roberts RO, Geda YE, Knopman DS, et al. The incidence of MCI differs by subtype and is higher in men: the Mayo Clinic Study of Aging. Neurology 2012;78: 342–51.
42. Petersen RC. Challenges of epidemiological studies of mild cognitive impairment. Alzheimer Dis Assoc Disord 2004;18:1–2.
43. Ganguli M, Dodge HH, Shen C, et al. Mild cognitive impairment, amnestic type: an epidemiologic study. Neurology 2004;63:115–21.
44. Ganguli M, Chang CC, Snitz BE, et al. Prevalence of mild cognitive impairment by multiple classifications: the Monongahela-Youghiogheny Healthy Aging Team (MYHAT) project. Am J Geriatr Psychiatry 2010;18:674–83.
45. Luck T, Riedel-Heller SG, Kaduszkiewicz H, et al. Mild cognitive impairment in general practice: age-specific prevalence and correlate results from the German study on ageing, cognition and dementia in primary care patients (Age-CoDe). Dement Geriatr Cogn Disord 2007;24:307–16.
46. Petersen RC, Roberts RO, Knopman DS, et al. Prevalence of mild cognitive impairment is higher in men. The Mayo Clinic Study of Aging. Neurology 2010;75:889–97.
47. Sattler C, Toro P, Schonknecht P, et al. Cognitive activity, education and socioeconomic status as preventive factors for mild cognitive impairment and Alzheimer's disease. Psychiatry Res 2012;196:90–5.
48. Lopez OL, Jagust WJ, DeKosky ST, et al. Prevalence and classification of mild cognitive impairment in the Cardiovascular Health Study Cognition Study: part 1. Arch Neurol 2003;60:1385–9.
49. Fisk JD, Merry HR, Rockwood K. Variations in case definition affect prevalence but not outcomes of mild cognitive impairment. Neurology 2003;61:1179–84.
50. Busse A, Hensel A, Guhne U, et al. Mild cognitive impairment: long-term course of four clinical subtypes. Neurology 2006;67:2176–85.
51. Das SK, Bose P, Biswas A, et al. An epidemiologic study of mild cognitive impairment in Kolkata, India. Neurology 2007;68:2019–26.
52. Larrieu S, Letenneur L, Orgogozo JM, et al. Incidence and outcome of mild cognitive impairment in a population-based prospective cohort. Neurology 2002;59:1594–9.
53. Tervo S, Kivipelto M, Hanninen T, et al. Incidence and risk factors for mild cognitive impairment: a population-based three-year follow-up study of cognitively healthy elderly subjects. Dement Geriatr Cogn Disord 2004;17:196–203.
54. Solfrizzi V, Panza F, Colacicco AM, et al. Vascular risk factors, incidence of MCI, and rates of progression to dementia. Neurology 2004;63:1882–91.
55. Palmer K, Backman L, Winblad B, et al. Mild cognitive impairment in the general population: occurrence and progression to Alzheimer disease. Am J Geriatr Psychiatry 2008;16:603–11.
56. Caracciolo B, Palmer K, Monastero R, et al. Occurrence of cognitive impairment and dementia in the community: a 9-year-long prospective study. Neurology 2008;70:1778–85.
57. Manly JJ, Tang MX, Schupf N, et al. Frequency and course of mild cognitive impairment in a multiethnic community. Ann Neurol 2008;63:494–506.
58. Ravaglia G, Forti P, Montesi F, et al. Mild cognitive impairment: epidemiology and dementia risk in an elderly Italian population. J Am Geriatr Soc 2008;56: 51–8.

59. Luck T, Luppa M, Briel S, et al. Mild cognitive impairment: incidence and risk factors: results of the Leipzig Longitudinal Study of the Aged. J Am Geriatr Soc 2010;58:1903–10.

60. Luck T, Riedel-Heller SG, Luppa M, et al. Risk factors for incident mild cognitive impairment—results from the German Study on Ageing, Cognition and Dementia in Primary Care Patients (AgeCoDe). Acta Psychiatr Scand 2010;121: 260–72.

61. Luck T, Luppa M, Wiese B, et al. Prediction of incident dementia: impact of impairment in instrumental activities of daily living and mild cognitive impairment—results from the German study on ageing, cognition, and dementia in primary care patients. Am J Geriatr Psychiatry 2012;20:943–54.

62. Mauri M, Sinforiani E, Zucchella C, et al. Progression to dementia in a population with amnestic mild cognitive impairment: clinical variables associated with conversion. Funct Neurol 2012;27:49–54.

63. Peters M, Rosenberg P, Steinberg M, et al. Neuropsychiatric symptoms as risk factors for progression from CIND to dementia: the cache county study. Am J Geriatr Psychiatry 2013. [Epub ahead of print]. http://dx.doi.org/10.1016/j.jagp.2013.01.049.

Cognitive and Emotional Dysfunction in Mild Cognitive Impairment

Suzanne Penna, PhD, ABPP[a,b]

KEYWORDS

- Cognition • Mild cognitive impairment • Measurement • Neuropsychiatric symptoms

KEY POINTS

- Both cognitive and emotional changes are seen in individuals with mild cognitive impairment (MCI). Given the heterogeneity of the disorder, there is no standard threshold constituting cognitive or functional impairment; rather, impairment is determined by clinical judgment. Several screening and functional measures are useful to assess for MCI; however, neuropsychological testing remains the definitive method of identifying and quantifying specific cognitive deficits.

- The most commonly seen cognitive impairments in MCI include impairments with memory, executive functioning, and language. Patterns of deficits are helpful in determining subtypes of MCI; with a broad division between those with and without memory impairment (amnestic MCI vs nonamnestic MCI), and a further division between individuals with only one cognitive domain affected versus those with multiple cognitive impairments. Different subtypes of MCI are associated with differing rates of conversion to dementia, and differing types of dementia.

- While all patients with MCI have cognitive impairments by definition, a substantial proportion of those with MCI also experience emotional changes, with rates of neuropsychiatric symptoms ranging from 35% to 85%.

- The most common neuropsychiatric symptoms seen in MCI include depression, anxiety, irritability, apathy, and agitation. Emotional changes are related to cognitive functioning in that a greater number and greater severity of neuropsychiatric symptoms were associated with poorer cognitive functioning, as well as greater impairment with activities of daily living (ADLs) and instrumental ADLs. Furthermore, a greater number of neuropsychiatric symptoms are associated with a higher rate of conversion to dementia.

- Depression, apathy, and anxiety are the most common neuropsychiatric symptoms associated with a conversion to dementia. There is some evidence that those with amnestic MCI are more likely to have depression than other subtypes, which is particularly true when there is also impairment in executive functioning.

Continued

Funding Sources: None.
Conflict of Interest: None.
[a] Atlanta Veteran's Affairs Medical Center, 1670 Clairmont Road, Atlanta, GA 30033, USA;
[b] Department of Rehabilitation Medicine, Emory University School of Medicine, Center for Rehabilitation Medicine, 1441 Clifton Road NE, Suite 150, Atlanta, GA 30022, USA
E-mail address: spenna@emory.edu

Continued

- It is unclear whether neuropsychiatric symptoms are reflective of pathologic changes in the brain, if they are the result of distress from changes in cognitive functioning, or if they are the cause of the cognitive impairment, as both depression and anxiety are associated with declines in memory and concentration. Thus the treatment of neuropsychiatric symptoms can serve to improve emotional functioning, but may also improve cognitive functioning.
- Unfortunately, there has been little research into the treatment of neuropsychiatric deficits in MCI, although studies have shown limited benefit from psychotropic medication in improving depression in those with Alzheimer dementia. There is some evidence that donepezil, which delayed the progression to dementia among depressed patients, may be an option for the treatment of neuropsychiatric symptoms in addition to traditional psychotropic medications.

The concept of mild cognitive impairment (MCI), both clinically and for research purposes, has been a useful one; however, significant heterogeneity has made characterization of the disorder difficult. This heterogeneity includes the presence of multiple causes underlying the condition, as well as significant comorbidities that may contribute to current symptoms. In addition, there continues to be a lack of consensus in the literature about how to identify and quantify deficits seen in individuals with MCI. The aim of this article is to explore neuropsychiatric deficits in individuals with MCI, including both cognitive and emotional changes seen in MCI.

The idea of a prodrome to Alzheimer dementia (AD) has been of clinical interest for many years.[1] However it was not until the landmark article in 1999 by Petersen and colleagues[2] that the concept of MCI was clearly identified and characterized both cross-sectionally and longitudinally. The importance of identifying this group of individuals is not just to identify a group at risk for dementia, but to also determine the rate of conversion to dementia, and identify factors that protect against further decline or increase the risk of progression (**Box 1**).

The study by Peterson and colleagues[2] examined 3 groups of individuals: the general medical population, those with MCI, and those diagnosed with AD at varying degrees of severity (Clinical Dementia Rating [CDR] 0.5 and 1.0, respectively). The investigators found that on neuropsychological measures of cognitive functioning there were no significant differences between the normal controls and MCI patients on most cognitive domains, with the exception of memory performance. On memory tasks, those with MCI had scores equivalent to those in the AD group. Also noted was a decline in performance for word retrieval, which may reflect either a naming

---

Box 1
Initial definition of mild cognitive impairment

- Memory complaint
- Normal activities of daily living
- Normal general cognitive functioning
- Abnormal memory for age
- Not demented

Data from Petersen R, Smith G, Waring S, et al. Mild cognitive impairment: clinical characterization and outcome. Arch Neurol 1999;56(3):303–8.

impairment or a semantic memory deficit. Conversion rates were 12% per year from MCI to AD, compared with conversion rates of 1% to 2% per year from normal controls to MCI/AD.[2]

CHANGES IN THE DEFINITION OF MCI

Since 1999 there has been a virtual explosion of research into MCI, which has revealed the construct to be significantly more heterogeneous than first reported.[3] In accordance with the diversity of research findings, the definition of MCI has adapted as well. Following the first meeting of the International Working Group on MCI in 2003 the general criteria for of MCI changed to "not normal, not demented."[4] This definition was further refined in 2011.[5] Specifically, this includes the criteria listed in **Box 2**.

COGNITIVE ASSESSMENT IN MCI

With regard to cognitive functioning, numerous critiques have been raised about MCI. Specifically there has been controversy regarding the degree or severity of cognitive impairment required for diagnosis, the variability among cognitive domains affected in MCI, and the degree of functional impairment seen in MCI.[4] In the literature, neuropsychological testing typically has been used to assess cognitive functioning in MCI.[6–10] Neuropsychological testing accurately distinguishes healthy controls from those with even mild cognitive impairment with more than 80% sensitivity and 90% specificity, and has been found to accurately predict progression to dementia.[11] While there is general agreement that broad areas of cognitive functioning need to be assessed to determine the presence and severity of cognitive impairment, there is no consensus regarding a specific test battery that is considered the gold standard for the diagnosis of MCI.

Typically, areas of cognitive functioning assessed by neuropsychologists include:

- Attention/working memory
- Psychomotor speed
- New learning and memory
- Language (expressive and receptive)
- Visual-spatial and constructional abilities
- Executive functioning (eg, verbal fluency, abstract reasoning, mental flexibility, deductive reasoning)

Box 2
National Institute on Aging–Alzheimer's Association criteria

1. Concern regarding a change in cognition (self or informant report)

2. Impairment in 1 or more cognitive domains (lower performance in one or more cognitive domains that is greater than would be expected for the patient's age and educational background)

3. Preservation of independence in functional abilities

4. Not demented—these cognitive changes should be sufficiently mild that there is no evidence of a significant impairment in social or occupational functioning

Adapted from Albert MS, DeKosky ST, Dickson D, et al. The diagnosis of mild cognitive impairment due to Alzheimer's disease: recommendations from the National Institute on Aging-Alzheimer's Association workgroups on diagnostic guidelines for Alzheimer's disease. Alzheimers Dement 2011;7(3):270–9.

CUTOFF SCORES INDICATING COGNITIVE IMPAIRMENT

There was some attempt to quantify subjective memory complaint in the initial Petersen and colleagues[2] longitudinal study, which was suggested as "generally 1.5 SD below average"; however, the investigators ultimately noted that the classifications described were clinically based, and the ultimate judgment of decline was based on that of the clinician. This approach was adopted by the participants of the International Working Group, who noted: "Individual slopes of decline in both functional and cognitive performance may be better measures than deficits assessed according to age-specific norms."[3]

Although different studies use different cutoff scores to define impairment on specific tests (ranging from −1.0 standard deviation [SD] to −2.0 SD[12]), MCI remains a clinical diagnosis, not a psychometric one.[2–5] Therefore if a patient has a performance 2 SD above the mean on the majority of neuropsychological tests administered and has memory performance in the average range (0 SD), this would represent a functional decline for this patient relative to his or her own performance, despite not falling within the psychometrically "impaired" range of performance.

USE OF FUNCTIONAL MEASURES TO ASSESS COGNITION

The CDR measure[13] is commonly used in research in dementia, but has also been used in the research literature on MCI. It is viewed as the gold-standard measure in pharmacologic studies of dementia medications. The CDR has primarily been used in the research literature and less so in clinical practice, largely due the time-intensive nature of the measure.[14] The CDR is a semistructured interview with the patient and an informant, and makes an overall level of impairment based on 6 cognitive categories: memory, orientation, judgment and problem solving, community affairs, home and hobbies, and personal care. This measure attempts to assess cognitive decline through functional impairment, rather than measure cognitive functioning objectively relative to population norms, which is done with neuropsychological testing.

Another commonly used questionnaire is the Functional Activities Questionnaire (FAQ),[14] an observer-rated report of a family member's ability to perform a multitude of functional activities (both activities of daily life [ADLs] and instrumental ADLs [IADLs]). Typically this scale is used in conjunction with other cognitive or screening measures when assessing MCI or dementia, as it provides good information about functional activities, but does not formally assess cognitive functioning.[15]

USE OF SCREENING MEASURES TO ASSESS COGNITION

Although neuropsychological assessment is considered the gold standard in assessing cognitive functioning, very often detailed neuropsychological testing is not available in medical clinics, particularly those not affiliated with a large medical center or in an underserved area. Alternatively, busy clinics that see a high number of geriatric patients often use brief cognitive screening measures to determine which patients to refer for more intensive neuropsychological testing. In either case, there are brief screening measures available to assess cognitive functioning, although it is important to emphasize that performance on these measures alone is not sufficient to diagnose the presence or absence of MCI. The most commonly used and best validated screening measures are presented here.[16]

The oldest, and likely still the most common measure of mental status, is the Mini Mental Status Examination (MMSE[17]), an examiner-administered cognitive screening originally developed to assess dementia. It consists of 30 questions assessing orientation, memory, attention, expressive language, and visual-spatial construction. The advantages of this measure are that it is quick to administer and that most practitioners are familiar with it. However, it is not an ideal measure for the assessment of MCI, most notably because of its emphasis on orientation, which is nearly always preserved in MCI. Not surprisingly, the MMSE has poor sensitivity for identifying MCI and discriminating it from either healthy controls or patients with dementia.[18] In addition, the MMSE is copyrighted and out of the public domain, which makes it a less cost-effective choice.

The screening measure with the greatest empiric validation is the Montreal Cognitive Assessment (MOCA[19]), which was designed specifically to screen for MCI. Similar to the MMSE, it is a 30-item measure that takes approximately 10 minutes to administer. It has a good balance across cognitive domains, with orientation, memory, attention/working memory, visual spatial skills, naming, and executive functioning. The MOCA has very good empirical support, with both good sensitivity (90% for MCI) and specificity (100% accuracy in identifying healthy controls).[19]

A more recent measure, the St Louis University Mental Status examination (SLUMS[20]), has been developed specifically for use in the veteran population. Again it is a 30-item questionnaire, which is a general cognitive screener. Validity studies have been promising, with diagnostic accuracies ranging from .927 to .941 (area under the curve) using receiver-operative characteristic curve analyses. The major disadvantage of the SLUMS is that it was developed for diagnosing Mild Neurocognitive Disorder (MNCD) according to the DSM-IV-TR (*Diagnostic and Statistical Manual of Mental Disorders* 4th edition, text revision) rather than MCI; thus there are some differences in the construct being measured in the SLUMS in comparison with the MOCA. Continued validity studies looking specifically at the MCI veteran population are still needed. Of note, although each measure has a maximum of 30 points, each measure has its own cutoff scores indicating impairment, so that scores out of 30 are not necessarily equivalent across measures (**Table 1**).

SUBTYPES OF MCI

Given the multiple purported causes underlying MCI (eg, neurodegenerative, vascular, metabolic, psychiatric), as well as the heterogeneity in cognitive performance on testing and variability in progression, MCI has been divided into subtypes based on the specificity of cognitive deficits noted. At present MCI is divided into 2 broad subtypes based on the presence or absence of memory dysfunction. If there is memory dysfunction, it is classified as amnestic MCI (aMCI). If there is no memory dysfunction,

Table 1					
Summary of cognitive screening measures commonly used for MCI					
Test	No. of Items	In the Public Domain?	Cognitive Domains	Sensitivity/ Specificity for MCI	Designed for Specific Population
MMSE	30	No	Heavy on orientation	Sensitivity 18% Specificity 87%	Screening for dementia
MOCA	30	Yes	Good distribution of cognitive domains	Sensitivity 90% Specificity 100%	Screening for MCI
SLUMS	30	Yes	Good distribution of cognitive domains	Diagnostic accuracy: .927 <12th grade .941 >12th grade	Screening for MNCD in veteran population

it is classified as nonamnestic MCI (naMCI). Groups are further delineated into either single or multiple cognitive domains affected.[3] Thus, the 4 subtypes are as follows: aMCI single domain; aMCI multidomain; naMCI, single domain; and naMCI multi domain. The advantage of this classification system is that it serves to organize the heterogeneous cognitive findings seen with MCI patients, and to explore both the etiology and trajectory of cognitive functioning in patients with these particular subtypes (**Fig. 1**).[12]

Rates of conversion of MCI to dementia typically fall between 12% and 15%.[5] However, this number accounts for the MCI population as a whole, not necessarily the rates of conversion in specific subtypes. In a recent longitudinal study, patients were classified into MCI subtypes and were followed over a year to determine rates of cognitive change.[12] Outcomes could be decline, stability, or improvement in cognitive functioning. The investigators used the CDR to assess for change over time, which focuses on cognitive decline in everyday functioning rather than objective measurement of cognitive functioning (eg, neuropsychological testing). The investigators found that the rates of progression to dementia across the MCI population were small, ranging from 0% to 3%. The multidomain aMCI group had the poorest outcome, with the highest percentage of patients experiencing cognitive decline (19.8%) and the lowest percentage experiencing cognitive improvement (6.3%). The single-domain naMCI group had the best outcome, with only 1.1% of patients experiencing a cognitive decline and 53.4% of the group experiencing cognitive improvement back to "normal" functioning. Of note, the majority of all MCI patients experienced stability in cognitive performance over the year, ranging from 28.6% (single-domain naMCI), to 44.1% (multidomain aMCI).

Two other recent longitudinal studies that examined the rates of progression by MCI subtypes also indicate that the type of MCI does influence rates of conversion to dementia. Norlund and colleagues[21] followed 209 participants with MCI using standard neuropsychological tests. Of the 175 seen for follow-up, 25% had progressed to dementia. Those with progression of cognitive deficits tended to be those with multidomain MCI. Those with aMCI multidomain (35 participants) were more likely to convert to dementia than those with naMCI multidomain (9 participants). In a similar study, participants were given a neuropsychological evaluation and followed over time.[6] The investigators found that those at greatest risk of progression to dementia were those in the aMCI multidomain group, rather than single-domain aMCI subjects. Specifically, they found that deficits in verbal memory, psychomotor speed, and executive functioning best predicted conversion to dementia.

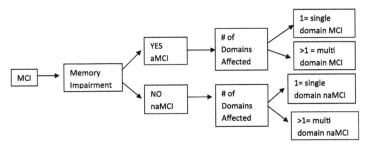

Fig. 1. MCI subtype classification. aMCI, amnestic MCI; naMCI, nonamnestic MCI. (*Data from* Winblad B, Palmer M, Kivipelto M, et al. Mild cognitive impairment—beyond controversies, toward a consensus: report of the International Working Group on Mild Cognitive Impairment. J Intern Med 2004;256:243.)

The amnestic and nonamnestic distinction has also been shown to be important in the types of dementia diagnosed when MCI does progress to dementia. Those with amnestic forms of MCI typically tend to progress to AD.[22] Those diagnosed with naMCI and have progression of cognitive impairment tend to be diagnosed with other forms of dementia (eg, vascular dementia or dementia with Lewy bodies[23]). The Goteborg MCI study[21] found that the cognitive profiles of patients who went on to develop AD or vascular dementia differed. While increased cognitive impairment across domains was associated with conversion to dementia in general, memory, visual-spatial, and language impairment preceded AD, and impairment of executive function, processing speed, and attention preceded vascular dementia.

IMPAIRMENT IN SPECIFIC COGNITIVE DOMAINS COMMONLY SEEN IN MCI

Deficits in all cognitive domains (eg, memory, visual-spatial skills, attention) have been reported in patients with MCI, which is not surprising given the heterogeneity of the disorder. Given the large body of research examining specific cognitive impairment in MCI, the focus is on the most common cognitive domains affected: memory, executive functioning, and language.

Memory

Given that the initial definition of MCI,[2] which had a requirement of memory impairment, and that the entire construct of MCI is hypothesized to be precursor to dementia, it is not surprising that one of the most commonly affected areas of cognitive functioning is that of memory.[2,6–8,10,12,21,24]

Memory is usually divided into 3 broad components in the neuropsychological literature: learning new information (encoding), recall of newly learned information after a delay, and recognition of newly learned information after a delay. Tests are further divided into verbal memory tasks or visual memory tasks. Declines have been seen on both types of memory tasks, although many studies collapsed all memory data into an overall composite score.[8,12]

Prospective memory, the ability to remember an event happening in the future (eg, remembering an upcoming doctor's appointment), has also been found to be impaired in patients with MCI.[25] The group of van den Berg conducted a meta-analytical review of studies of prospective memory in both MCI and dementia from 1990 to 2011. Of the 7 studies examining prospective memory in MCI, all found declines in prospective memory, and there was no significant difference between event-based or time-based prospective memory. The investigators also found moderate correlations in test performance between measures of prospective memory and measures of retrospective memory, as well as correlations between prospective memory and executive functioning.[25]

A recent study has looked at memory impairment in aMCI in a novel way by examining the ability of patients with MCI to benefit from practice effects.[10] Typically the time between repeated neuropsychological assessments is approximately a year, given concerns about practice effects (eg, exposure to cognitive tests produces improvement on repeat testing owing to familiarity with the measures). In this study the investigators performed a baseline neuropsychological assessment, then retested the subjects a week later. Groups were divided into healthy controls, aMCI with strong practice effects, and aMCI with minimal practice effects. A year later patients were retested, and those with minimal practice effects performed significantly worse than aMCI subjects with good practice effects and normal controls on tasks of memory as well as language and overall cognition.

Executive Functioning

Executive functioning is a broad construct that assesses many aspects of cognition and behavior thought to be mediated by the prefrontal cortex, including planning, reasoning, judgment, mental flexibility, organization, initiation, and inhibition of behavior.[26] A study by Brandt and colleagues[9] looked at specific aspects of executive functioning that appear to be affected in MCI. Using principal-components analysis, the 17 executive functioning measures used in the study were divided into 3 broad domains: planning/problem solving, working memory, and judgment. The investigators found that both planning/problem solving and working memory deficits were commonly seen in MCI patients, with judgment being relatively persevered. Specifically, multiple-domain MCI patients had more severe impairments in executive functioning than those in single-domain subtypes.

Two longitudinal studies have found that executive dysfunction is predictive of later cognitive decline. Blacker and colleagues[8] attempted to determine which neuropsychological measures were associated with cognitive decline, looking at 2 groups: healthy controls and those diagnosed with MCI. These groups were followed over 5 years. In healthy controls, only difficulties on measures of memory were associated with cognitive decline over time. For those in the MCI group, both memory impairment and executive functioning were significant predictors of conversion to dementia. The second study followed a group of participants with MCI across 4 years and looked at their performance on 18 different measures of executive functioning.[27] Over the 4-year period, 35% of the population had a cognitive decline, with patients diagnosed with multi-domain MCI (both amnestic and nonamnestic) being associated with higher rates of progression. Eight of the 18 measures were associated with cognitive decline, including ones looking at mental flexibility and response inhibition.

Language

Language is typically viewed in 2 broad domains, language expression and language comprehension. In both MCI and AD, deficits are far more commonly seen with language expression, particularly naming and language fluency (although many conceptualize fluency more as an executive functioning measure than as a language measure). Naming seems to be particularly vulnerable in this population, and it has been hypothesized that the deficits in naming reflect an impairment of semantic knowledge rather than problems with lexical access.[28] Ahmed and colleagues[29] examined naming with patients with diagnosed aMCI relative to peers. The results indicated that patients with aMCI performed significantly worse relative to controls on all measures of naming, with specific difficulty in naming famous faces. Another study examined the neuropsychological performance on 112 patients with MCI compared with controls, and found that the clearest differences between groups were seen on language tests, followed by executive measures and then memory measures.[30] However, a study from the Mayo group found that although initial performance on a naming test was associated with increased risk for the development of AD, this risk was not nearly as significant as impaired performance on memory measures, specifically delayed recall.[31]

CHANGES IN PSYCHOLOGICAL/EMOTIONAL FUNCTIONING IN MCI
Population Studies

Although much of the research in MCI has focused on the cognitive effects of the syndrome, there has been a more recent effort to determine whether emotional effects are also seen. The initial comprehensive assessment of psychiatric disturbance in MCI was published by Lykestos and colleagues[32] in 2002. To date, it is one of only two population-based studies of neuropsychiatric sequelae in MCI. The study was one aspect of a larger multicenter, longitudinal study, the Cardiovascular Health Study. A total of 3608 participants were evaluated over 10 years in 4 United States counties, with a resultant 320 being diagnosed with MCI and 362 diagnosed with dementia. All participants completed the Neuropsychiatric Inventory (NPI), a structured interview assessing 12 psychiatric symptoms associated with cognitive disorders that utilizes both informant knowledge and observable symptoms and behaviors. Both frequency and severity scores are generated on each of the 12 domains and multiplied to obtain a total domain score, ranging from 0 to 20. A score greater than 4 on any single domain is considered clinically significant (**Box 3**).[33]

Forty-three percent of the participants diagnosed with MCI had evidence of neuropsychiatric symptoms over the past month, with 29% rated as clinically significant. The most common symptoms included depression, apathy, and irritability. Seventy-five percent of the participants diagnosed with dementia had evidence of neuropsychiatric symptoms, with 62% rated as clinically significant. The most common symptoms in the dementia group included apathy, depression, and agitation/aggression. Although the healthy elderly were not directly assessed in the study, the results were compared with findings from the Cache County Study,[34] which studied NPI symptoms from 652 cognitively healthy elderly patients ages 65 years and up. There was a significant difference between the MCI group and the cognitively healthy group for agitation/aggression, depression, apathy, irritability, and aberrant motor behavior. There were no differences between the MCI and cognitively healthy group for all other NPI domains. The investigators concluded that in parallel with cognitive changes in MCI, emotional changes in MCI represent a continuum, with greater cognitive impairment being associated with more significant emotional disturbance (and vice versa) (**Tables 2** and **3**).

The second population-based study examining the prevalence of neuropsychiatric symptoms in MCI came from the Mayo Clinic Study of Aging.[35] The investigators used a cross-sectional case-control study comparing MCI patients with healthy elderly with intact cognition. This study addressed the lack of a control group in the Cardiovascular Health Study by obtaining all participants from the same population. The participants were selected using random stratified sampling from a target population of nearly 10,000 people. Neurologic, cognitive, and psychiatric data were obtained, and individuals were grouped into either a healthy elderly control or MCI group by an expert consensus panel. The resulting pool of study participants consisted of 329 individuals diagnosed with MCI and 1640 classified as healthy controls. Participants with dementia were not included in the study. A short form of the NPI, the Neuropsychiatric Inventory Questionnaire (NPI-Q[36]), was used to assess the presence and severity of psychiatric symptoms. Between-group differences in age, gender, and education were statically controlled.

Box 3
NPI symptom domains

Delusions	Hallucinations	Agitation/aggression
Depression	Anxiety	Euphoria
Apathy	Disinhibition	Irritability
Sleep	Eating	Aberrant motor behavior

Frequency Score (Range 0–4) × Severity Score (Range 0–5) = Domain Score

Overall, approximately 25% of healthy controls had at least 1 neuropsychiatric symptom, compared with 50% of the MCI group. In general, there were higher rates of nonpsychotic symptoms (eg, depression, anxiety) than psychotic symptoms (delusions, hallucinations) in both groups, with psychotic symptoms occurring very rarely. Similar to the results of the Cardiovascular Health Study, the highest frequency of symptoms in MCI were depression, apathy, and irritability. Statically significant differences between MCI and control groups were also seen on symptoms of agitation and anxiety.

Comparison of results between the Mayo Clinic Study of Aging and Cardiovascular Health Study				
	MCI		Healthy Controls	
	Mayo	**CHS**	**Mayo**	**CHS Cache County Data**
Overall prevalence of neuropsychiatric symptoms	50%	43%	25%	Not reported
Rates of specific neuropsychiatric symptoms	Depression (27%) Apathy (18.5%) Irritability (19.4%)	Depression (20%) Apathy (15%) Irritability (15%)	Depression (11.5%) Apathy (4.8%) Irritability (7.6%)	Depression (7.2%) Apathy (3.2%) Irritability (4.6%)

The investigators also looked at rates of neuropsychiatric symptoms based on subtype of MCI. Those with aMCI reported greater symptoms of apathy, agitation, and irritability than those with naMCI. Those with naMCI reported greater symptoms of depression and anxiety.

Neuropsychiatric symptom differences between anamnestic and nonanamnestic MCI in the Mayo Study		
	aMCI	**naMCI**
Apathy	48 (20.7%)[a]	11 (12.6%)
Agitation	22 (9.5%)[a]	7 (8%)
Irritability	46 (19.8%)[a]	16 (18.4%)
Anxiety	32 (13.8%)	13 (14.9%)[b]
Depression	60 (25.9)	26 (29.9%)[b]

[a] Statistically significant difference in aMCI.
[b] Statistically significant difference in naMCI.

LITERATURE REVIEWS OF EMOTIONAL CHANGES IN MCI

Apostolova and Cummings[37] reviewed existing literature on neuropsychiatric symptoms in MCI, to determine whether psychiatric disturbance could be used as a biomarker for impending dementia. The investigators performed a PubMed search on all English-language studies of neuropsychiatric symptoms in MCI before December 2006. Search criteria included a sample size of at least 20 participants, a clear description of MCI diagnostic criteria used, and a clear description of the methodology of data collection regarding behavioral/psychotic data. Twenty-one studies

Table 2
Findings from the cardiovascular health study

	MCI (n = 320)	Dementia (n = 362)
Percentage reporting symptoms over the past month	43	75
Percentage of symptoms that met clinical significance	29	62
Most common symptoms reported	Depression Apathy Irritability	Apathy Depression Agitation/aggression

were identified using these criteria. Seven were population based, 12 were from tertiary memory disorder centers, and 1 was a clinical trial. Ten studies were longitudinal and 11 used cross-sectional data. Results indicated that neuropsychiatric symptoms are common in MCI, with rates ranging from 35% to 75%. The most common consistently reported symptoms include depression, apathy, irritability, and anxiety, despite widely variable study designs, sample sizes, behavioral assessment, and MCI diagnostic criteria used. The least common symptoms include euphoria, hallucinations, disinhibition, and aberrant motor behavior.

A second literature review was published by Monastero and colleagues,[38] using search criteria similar to those of Apostolova and Cummings. This study included a PubMed review of articles including a definition of MCI, specific cognitive testing, the use of standardized instruments to assess neuropsychiatric symptoms, and a sample size of at least 40. Using these criteria 27 studies were identified and reviewed; 12 were hospital based, 2 were multicenter clinical trials, 11 were population-based studies, and 1 was a study of elderly clergy throughout the United States. Their review found prevalence rates of neuropsychiatric symptoms in MCI ranging from 35% to 85%. There were higher rates of neuropsychiatric symptoms in hospital-based studies than in population-based studies, which was attributed to selection bias. In addition, differences in age, gender, and inclusion/exclusion criteria significantly affected prevalence rates of psychiatric symptoms. Again, the most commonly reported neuropsychiatric symptoms included depression, anxiety, irritability, apathy, and agitation. Psychotic symptoms and elation were relatively rare.

Table 3
Findings from the cardiovascular health study

	MCI vs Healthy Controls
Symptoms with significant difference between groups	Agitation/aggression Depression Apathy Aberrant motor behavior
Symptoms with no significant difference between groups	Anxiety Disinhibition Irritability Delusions Hallucinations Euphoria Sleep Eating

Relation Between Emotional Dysfunction and Cognitive Dysfunction

Investigators on the InDDEX trial examined the relation between emotional distress and cognitive performance, and found that those with clinically significant neuropsychiatric symptoms on the NPI did more poorly on measures of global cognitive functioning and measures of functional independence.[39] Similarly, Hudon and colleagues[40] examined the effect of depression on cognitive functioning in individuals with aMCI. Whereas there were no differences in memory performance between depressed and nondepressed individuals, there was a significant difference in performance on executive functioning, with those experiencing depression having poorer scores. Another population-based study found that the presence of any neuropsychiatric symptoms were associated with impairments in both IADLs and ADLs.[41]

NEUROPSYCHIATRIC SYMPTOMS ASSOCIATED WITH MCI SUBTYPES

Rosenberg and colleagues[42] examined neuropsychiatric symptoms among various subtypes of MCI, including aMCI, naMCI, and those with those with and without executive dysfunction. Results indicated no differences in prevalence of neuropsychiatric symptoms between aMCI and naMCI groups. However, when examining differences between groups with and without impairment of executive functioning, the investigators found that those with executive dysfunction had significantly greater severity of depression and anxiety than those without deficits in executive functioning. This finding is similar to that of Hudon and colleagues[40] as noted in the previous section. In a longitudinal study by Edwards and colleagues,[43] 521 patients with MCI were divided into subtypes and assessed for the presence and severity of neuropsychiatric symptoms. Results indicated that overall, patients with greater than 4 neuropsychiatric symptoms (using DSM-III criteria) had 2.5 times the odds of developing dementia over time than patients with fewer than 3 neuropsychiatric symptoms. Those with greater than 4 neuropsychiatric symptoms were slightly more likely to have a diagnosis of amnestic MCI (81% vs 71%, $P = .03$). Also, those with aMCI were likely to report symptoms of depression than were other subtypes. Rozzini and colleagues[7] found that those with naMCI were more likely to report hallucinations and sleep disorders than were those with aMCI. There were no other differences in prevalence of neuropsychiatric symptoms reported between groups.

NEUROPSYCHIATRIC SYMPTOMS AND RISK FOR PROGRESSION TO DEMENTIA

There has been speculation that aMCI is a precursor to AD, and that naMCI is a precursor to other types of dementia (eg, Lewy body dementia or frontotemporal dementia).[5,44] The Rozzini study already cited[7] appears to lend some support to this, given the differing types of psychiatric symptoms reported between subtypes, although this seems to be the only study looking at MCI subtypes that has found these differences.

As mentioned earlier, Edwards and colleagues[43] have found that those with greater than 4 neuropsychiatric symptoms were at 2.5 times greater risk of developing dementia than those with fewer than 3 symptoms. Several other studies have supported the hypothesis that number and severity of neuropsychiatric symptoms, particularly depression, apathy, and anxiety, were associated with an increased risk of conversion to dementia.[45–49] Modrego and Ferrandez[48] found that patients with MCI and neuropsychiatric symptoms who had a poor response to antidepressant therapy were at increased risk for the development of dementia.[49] Apathy has also been examined as a potential precursor to dementia.[50] In a study of 216 patients with aMCI, 86 initially presented with at least 1 symptom of apathy. Of those, 15% converted to AD after a year, compared with 6.9% of the aMCI patients who did not endorse apathy.

Other studies have found no relation between depression and progression from MCI to dementia. The results of the Italian Longitudinal Study on Aging (ILSA) found no evidence for depression as a predictor of progression from MCI to dementia, nor was there any indication that baseline symptoms of depression were a risk factor for the later development of MCI.[51,52] In addition, a longitudinal study of aging Catholic priests in the United States produced similar results.[53]

TREATMENT OF NEUROPSYCHIATRIC IMPAIRMENTS IN MCI

At this point it is unclear if neuropsychiatric symptoms may be reflective of pathologic changes in the brain, or whether they are the result of distress from changes in cognitive functioning.[38] Furthermore, many times a primary psychiatric disorder, such as depression or anxiety, may actually be the cause of perceived changes in cognitive functioning, as impairments with concentration and memory are commonly reported in these disorders across the life span. Symptoms of depression and anxiety may be interpreted as cognitive impairment, but remit with successful treatment of the disorder. As emotional symptoms have a strong influence on cognitive functioning, appropriate treatment of psychiatric symptoms may serve to reverse the diagnosis.[38,54]

There is a paucity of literature examining response to psychotropic medication in patients with MCI who have neuropsychiatric symptoms. Recent research has found that psychotropic medication is not particularly effective in the treatment of depression in AD, although psychosocial intervention targeted at caregivers did have a beneficial effect.[55] Li and colleagues[56] longitudinally followed controls and patients with MCI, AD, and vascular dementia, and found that the patients with vascular dementia and MCI with depression were most refractory to antidepressant medications. However, of the 3 clinical groups, those with MCI had the lowest rates of depression. An additional study of 39 patients with comorbid MCI and depression found a 65% response rate to treatment with sertraline. There was no difference in subtype of MCI among responders to treatment.[57] Cognitive improvement was not observed in responders, apart from one measure of processing speed.

However, one study indicated that while depression increases the risk of conversion from MCI to AD, treatment with donepezil delayed progression to dementia among depressed MCI patients.[58] It is possible that although depression is more resistant to selective serotonin-reuptake inhibitor therapy in patients with MCI or dementia, the effect of depression can be modulated by acetylcholinesterase (ACh)-inhibitor medications. Because neuropsychiatric symptoms in patients with MCI do not appear to respond particularly well to traditional psychiatric medications, research into alternative medications (eg, ACh inhibitors) and psychotherapeutic approaches would greatly benefit the MCI population.

SUMMARY

Both cognitive and emotional changes are seen in individuals with MCI. Given the heterogeneity of the disorder, there is no standard threshold constituting cognitive or functional impairment; rather, impairment is determined by clinical judgment. Several screening and functional measures are useful for assessing MCI, although neuropsychological testing remains the definitive method for identifying and quantifying specific cognitive deficits. The most commonly seen cognitive impairments in MCI are impairments of memory, executive functioning, and language. Patterns of deficits are helpful in determining subtypes of MCI; with a broad division between those with and without memory impairment (aMCI vs naMCI), and a further division between individuals with only 1 affected cognitive domain versus those with multiple cognitive impairments. Different subtypes of MCI are associated with differing rates of conversion to dementia, and differing types of dementia.

While all patients with MCI have cognitive impairments by definition, a substantial proportion of those with MCI also experience emotional changes, with rates of neuropsychiatric symptoms ranging from 35% to 85%. The most common neuropsychiatric symptoms seen in MCI include depression, anxiety, irritability, apathy, and agitation. Emotional changes are related to cognitive functioning in that both more severe and a greater number of neuropsychiatric symptoms were associated with poorer cognitive functioning, as well as greater impairment of IADLs and ADLs. Furthermore, a greater number of neuropsychiatric symptoms are associated with a higher rate of conversion to dementia. Depression, apathy, and anxiety are the most common neuropsychiatric symptoms associated with a conversion to dementia. There is some evidence that those with aMCI are more likely to have depression than other subtypes, which is particularly true when there is also impairment of executive functioning.[42] One study found that sleep disorders and hallucinations were more commonly seen in naMCI[7]; otherwise no distinctions between MCI subtypes and emotional symptoms have been reported. It is unclear as to whether neuropsychiatric symptoms are reflective of pathologic changes in the brain, if they are the result of distress from changes in cognitive functioning, or whether they are the cause of the cognitive impairment, as both depression and anxiety are associated with declines in memory and concentration. Thus, treatment of neuropsychiatric symptoms can serve to improve emotional functioning, but may also improve cognitive functioning. Unfortunately, there has been little research into the treatment of neuropsychiatric deficits in MCI, although studies have shown limited benefit from psychotropic medication in improving depression in those with AD. There is some evidence that donepezil delayed progression to dementia among depressed patients, which suggests another option for the treatment of neuropsychiatric symptoms apart from traditional psychotropic medications. However, there is a need for more research in this area, particularly looking at MCI specifically rather than at patients with dementia.

REFERENCES

1. Kral VA. Senescent forgetfulness: benign and malignant. Can Med Assoc J 1962;86:257–60.
2. Petersen R, Smith G, Waring S, et al. Mild cognitive impairment: clinical characterization and outcome. Arch Neurol 1999;56(3):303–8.
3. Winblad B, Palmer M, Kivipelto M, et al. Mild cognitive impairment—beyond controversies, towards a consensus: report of the International Working Group on Mild Cognitive Impairment. J Intern Med 2004;256:240–6.
4. Albert MS, DeKosky ST, Dickson D, et al. The diagnosis of mild cognitive impairment due to Alzheimer's disease: recommendations from the National Institute on Aging-Alzheimer's Association workgroups on diagnostic guidelines for Alzheimer's disease. Alzheimers Dement 2011;7(3):270–9.
5. Petersen R, Rosebud O, Roberts M, et al. Mild cognitive impairment: ten years later. Arch Neurol 2009;66(12):1447–55.
6. Tabert M, Manly J, Liu X, et al. Neuropsychological prediction of conversion to Alzheimer's disease in patient with mild cognitive impairment. Arch Gen Psychiatry 2006;63(8):916–24.

7. Rozzini L, Chilovi B, Conti M, et al. Conversion of amnestic mild cognitive impairment to dementia of Alzheimer type is independent to memory deterioration. Int J Geriatr Psychiatry 2007;22(12):1217–22.

8. Blacker D, Lee H, Muzikansky A, et al. Neuropsychological measures in normal individuals that predict subsequent cognitive decline. Arch Neurol 2007;64(6): 862–71.

9. Brandt J, Aretouli E, Neijstrom E, et al. Selectivity of executive function deficits in mild cognitive impairment. Neuropsychology 2009;23(5):607–18.

10. Duff K, Lykestos C, Beglinger L, et al. Practice effects predict cognitive outcome in amnestic mild cognitive impairment. Am J Geriatr Psychiatry 2011;19:932–9.

11. Jacova C, Kertesz A, Blair M, et al. Neuropsychological testing and assessment for dementia. Alzheimers Dement 2007;3:299–317.

12. Ganguli M, Snitz B, Saxton J, et al. Outcomes of mild cognitive impairment by definition. Arch Neurol 2011;68(6):761–7.

13. Morris J. The Clinical Dementia Rating (CDR); current version and scoring rules. Neurology 1993;43(11):2412–4.

14. Morris J. Clinical dementia rating: a reliable and valid diagnostic and staging measure for dementia of the Alzheimer type. Int Psychogeriatr 1997;9:173–6.

15. Pfeffer R, Kurosaki T, Harrah C, et al. Measurement of functional activities in older adults in the community. J Gerontol 1982;37(3):323–9.

16. Lonie J, Tierney K, Ebmeier K. Screening for mild cognitive impairment: a systematic review. Int J Geriatr Psychiatry 2009;24:902–15.

17. Folstein M, Folstein S, McHugh P. 'Mini-mental state.' A practical method for grading the cognitive state of patients for the clinician. J Psychiatr Res 1975;2:189–98.

18. Mitchel A. A meta-analysis of the accuracy of the mini-mental state examination in the detection of dementia and mild cognitive impairment. J Psychiatr Res 2009;43:411–31.

19. Nasreddine Z, Phillips N, Bedirian V, et al. The Montreal Cognitive Assessment: a brief screening tool for mild cognitive impairment. J Am Geriatr Soc 2005;53: 695–9.

20. Tariq S, Chibnall J, Perry M, et al. Comparison of the Saint Louis University mental status examination and the mini-mental state examination for detecting dementia and mild neurocognitive disorder—a pilot study. Am J Geriatr Psychiatry 2006;14(11):900–10.

21. Norlund A, Ralstad S, Klang O, et al. Two-year outcome of MCI subtypes and aetiologies in the Goteborg MCI study. J Neurol Neurosurg Psychiatry 2010; 81(5):541–6.

22. Roberts R, Geda Y, Knopman D, et al. The Mayo Clinic Study of Aging: design and sampling, participation, baseline measures and sample characteristics. Neuroepidemiology 2008;30:58–69.

23. Molano J, Boeve B, Ferman T, et al. Mild cognitive impairment associated with limbic and neocortical Lewy body disease: a clincopathological study. Brain 2010;133:540–56.

24. Visser P, Scheltens P, Verhey F, et al. Medial temporal lobe atrophy and memory dysfunction as predictors for dementia in subjects with mild cognitive impairment. J Neurol 1999;246:477–85.

25. Van der Berg E, Kant N, Postman A. Remember to buy milk on the way home! A meta-analytic review of prospective memory in mild cognitive impairment and dementia. J Int Neuropsychol Soc 2012;18(4):706–16.

26. Malloy P, Cohen R, Jenkins M, et al. Frontal lobe function and dysfunction. In: Synder P, Nussbaum P, Robins D, editors. Clinical neuropsychology: a pocket

guide for assessment. 2nd edition. Washington, DC: American Psychological Association; 2006. p. 607–25.

27. Aretouli E, Tsilidis K, Brandt J. Four-year outcome of mild cognitive impairment: the contribution of executive dysfunction. Neuropsychology 2013;27(1):95–106.

28. Greene J, Hodges J. Identification of famous faces and famous names in early Alzheimer's disease: relationship to anterograde episodic and general semantic memory. Brain 1996;119(1):111–28.

29. Ahmed S, Arnold R, Thompson S, et al. Naming of objects, faces and buildings in mild cognitive impairment. Cortex 2008;48:746–52.

30. Nordlund A, Rolstad S, Hellstrom P, et al. The Goteborg MCI study: mild cognitive impairment is a heterogeneous condition. J Neurol Neurosurg Psychiatry 2005;76:1485–90.

31. Testa J, Ivnik R, Boeve B, et al. Confrontation naming does not add incremental diagnostic utility in MCI and Alzheimer's disease. J Int Neuropsychol Soc 2004; 10:504–12.

32. Lykestos C, Lopez O, Jones B, et al. Prevalence of neuropsychiatric symptoms in dementia and mild cognitive impairment: results from the Cardiovascular Health Study. JAMA 2002;288(121):11475–83.

33. Cummings J, Mega M, Gray K, et al. The Neuropsychiatric Inventory: comprehensive assessment of psychopathology in dementia. Neurology 1994;44: 2308–14.

34. Lystestos C, Steinberg M, Tschantz J, et al. Mental and neuropsychiatric symptoms in dementia: findings from the Cache County on Memory in Aging. Am J Psychiatry 2000;157:708–14.

35. Geda Y, Roberts R, Knopman D, et al. Prevalence of neuropsychiatric symptoms in mild cognitive impairment and normal cognitive aging. Arch Gen Psychiatry 2008;65(10):1193–8.

36. Kaufer D, Cummings J, Ketchel P, et al. Validation of the NPI-Q, a brief clinical form of the Neuropsychiatric Inventory. J Neuropsychiatry Clin Neurosci 2000; 12(2):233–9.

37. Apostolova L, Cummings J. Neuropsychiatric manifestations in mild cognitive impairment: a systematic review of the literature. Dement Geriatr Cogn Disord 2008;25:115–26.

38. Monastero R, Mangialasche F, Camarda C, et al. A systematic review of neuropsychiatric symptoms in mild cognitive impairment. J Alzheimers Dis 2009;18: 11–30.

39. Feldman H, Scheltens P, Scarpini E, et al. Behavioral symptoms in mild cognitive impairment. Neurology 2004;62:1199–201.

40. Hudon C, Belleville S, Gauthier S. The association between depressive and cognitive symptoms in amnestic mild cognitive impairment. Int Psychogeriatr 2008;20:710–23.

41. Chan D, Kasper J, Black B, et al. Prevalence and correlates of behavioral and psychiatric symptoms in community-dwelling elders with dementia or mild cognitive impairment: the Memory and Medical Care study. Int J Geriatr Psychiatry 2003;18:174–82.

42. Rosenberg P, Mielke M, Appleby B, et al. Neuropsychiatric symptoms in MCI subtypes: the importance of executive dysfunction. Int J Geriatr Psychiatry 2011;26(4):364–72.

43. Edwards E, Spira A, Barnes D, et al. Neuropsychiatric symptoms in mild cognitive impairment: differences by subtype and progression to dementia. Int J Geriatr Psychiatry 2009;24(7):716–22.

44. Mariani E, Monastero R, Mecocci P. Mild cognitive impairment: a systematic review. J Alzheimers Dis 2007;12:23–35.
45. Stepaniuk J, Ritchie L, Tuokko H. Neuropsychiatric impairments as predictors of mild cognitive impairment, dementia, and Alzheimer's disease. Am J Alzheimers Dis Other Demen 2009;23:326–33.
46. Gabryelewicz T, Styczynska M, Luczywek E, et al. The rate of conversion of mild cognitive impairment to dementia: predictive role of depression. Int J Geriatr Psychiatry 2007;22(6):563–7.
47. Houde M, Bergman H, Whithead V, et al. A predictive depression pattern in mild cognitive impairment. Int J Geriatr Psychiatry 2008;23:1028–33.
48. Modrego P, Ferrandez J. Depression in patients with mild cognitive impairment increases the risk of developing dementia of Alzheimer type: a prospective cohort study. Arch Neurol 2004;61:1290–3.
49. Panza F, Frisardi V, Capurso C, et al. Late life depression, mild cognitive impairment, and dementia: a possible continuum? Am J Geriatr Psychiatry 2010;18(2): 98–116.
50. Robert P, Berr C, Volteau M, et al. Apathy in patients with mild cognitive impairment and the risk of developing dementia of Alzheimer's disease: a one-year follow-up study. Clin Neurol Neurosurg 2006;108:733–6.
51. Panza F, D'Introno A, Colacicco A, et al. Depressive symptoms, vascular risk factors and mild cognitive impairment. The Italian longitudinal study on aging. Dement Geriatr Cogn Disord 2008;25:336–46.
52. Panza F, Capurso C, D'Introno A, et al. Impact of depressive symptoms on the rate of progression to dementia in patients affected by mild cognitive impairment. The Italian longitudinal study on aging. Int J Geriatr Psychiatry 2008;23: 726–34.
53. Wilson R, Arnold S, Beck T, et al. Change in depressive symptom during the prodromal phase of Alzheimer disease. Arch Gen Psychiatry 2008;65:439–45.
54. Palmer K, Wang H, Backman L, et al. Differential evolution of cognitive impairment in nondemented older persons: results from the Kungsholmen Project. Am J Psychiatry 2002;159:436–42.
55. Rosenberg P, Drye L, Martin B, et al, The DIADS-2 Research Group. Sertraline for the treatment of depression in Alzheimer's disease. Am J Geriatr Psychiatry 2010;18(2):136–45.
56. Li Y, Meyer J, Thornby J. Longitudinal follow-up of depressive symptom among normal versus cognitively impaired elderly. Int J Geriatr Psychiatry 2001;16: 718–27.
57. Devannand D, Pelton G, Marston K, et al. Sertraline treatment of elderly patients with depression and cognitive impairment. Int J Geriatr Psychiatry 2003;18: 123–30.
58. Lu P, Edland S, Teng E, et al. Donepezil delays progression to AD in MCI subjects with depressive symptoms. Neurology 2009;72(24):2115–21.

Clinical Evaluation of Early Cognitive Symptoms

J. Riley McCarten, MD[a,b]

KEYWORDS

- Cognitive • Dementia • Memory • Executive • Alzheimer

KEY POINTS

- An informant (spouse, family member) who knows the patient well is essential to obtaining the history.
- The onset, course, and nature of symptoms are the most important determinants of the etiology of cognitive impairment.
- Standard mental status tests are useful in clinic, but none are diagnostic. The physician must have a good understanding of basic cognitive functions.
- Targeting high-yield aspects of the neurologic examination allows an efficient evaluation and contributes to the differential diagnosis.
- The patient should be present throughout the process of taking the history and providing a diagnosis.

INTRODUCTION

Evaluating symptoms of cognitive impairment shares the basic elements of evaluating symptoms related to other complaints. The onset, course, and nature of symptoms are key to the history and dictate the essential features of the examination. Although it is important to allow patients/informants to describe symptoms in their own words, it is essential that the physician clearly understands the symptoms from a medical perspective. Furthermore, it is crucial that important questions relevant to the etiology of symptoms are addressed. Just as for headache, chest pain, nausea, or dizziness, the investigation of cognitive symptoms needs a combination of open-ended and directed questions to elicit the critical features of the history.

Funding Sources: VA Cooperative Studies Program, VA HSR&D, NIH, Minnesota Veterans Medical Research & Education Foundation.
Conflicts of Interest: None.
[a] Department of Neurology, University of Minnesota Medical School, 420 Delaware Street SE, Minneapolis, MN 55455, USA; [b] Geriatric Research, Education and Clinical Center (GRECC), Veterans Affairs Health Care System, One Veterans Drive, Minneapolis, MN 55417, USA
E-mail address: mccar034@umn.edu

Evaluating cognitive symptoms, however, does pose challenges not common to other symptoms. Cognitive functions are by far the most complex of biological functions. Symptoms of neocortical dysfunction can be challenging for experts to describe, much less the layperson. Patients often do not recognize the nature or severity of cognitive symptoms, and may be defensive. Family and/or providers may minimize the patient's symptoms for a variety of reasons: Challenging the integrity of one's cognitive function may seem disrespectful, particularly if the investigation is uninvited. Cognitive symptoms increase with age and may be seen as an inevitable part of aging, are difficult to assess, and the evaluation may be unsatisfying. Lastly and most importantly, even moderately demented patients, several years into a progressive dementia, may appear cognitively normal during a typical office visit. This fact cannot be overstated. Primary care physicians overlook cognitive impairment far too often.[1,2]

Though challenging, a structured approach to the evaluation of cognitive symptoms should provide the information needed to make informed clinical decisions in the best interest of patients, caregivers, and providers.

The foregoing describes the clinical evaluation in a medically stable outpatient. The diagnosis of a progressive, irreversible cognitive disorder should not be made in an acutely ill or stressed older adult. Conversely, awareness of underlying cognitive impairment can prepare providers, family, and the patient for the commonly seen exacerbation of cognitive symptoms when illness and stress do occur.

THE INTERVIEW
Overview

When the patient presents with cognitive complaints, or when problems are suspected during the course of the interview or examination, it is best to have a knowledgable informant available. Often this informant is in the waiting room. Because cognitive problems are so common in the elderly, it is reasonable to ask any unaccompanied older patient if he or she came with anyone, and if it would be permissible for that person to join the interview. The request is rarely denied.

If the patient is truly alone and cognitive symptoms are suspected, do not waste time with a potentially unreliable history. Rather, move directly to mental-status testing. If deficits are identified, the time saved can be used to identify an informant and review the history. Problems identified in the course of a visit not specifically for cognitive symptoms usually will require a separate appointment.

Symptoms of cognitive impairment often are intertwined with complex psychosocial issues. When dementia is clearly present, cognitive impairment is readily recognized as a contributing factor. When cognitive impairment is mild or questionable, it may be difficult to identify the difference between symptoms caused by brain disease and those related to anxiety, depression, medications, or situational factors. Patients and families often have their own ideas about cause, and may offer elaborate but tangential examples to support their viewpoints. Conversely, patients or, more often, families may be reluctant to discuss sensitive issues. It is important, therefore, that the physician establish the ground rules for the interview process to promote an efficient and thorough assessment.

Setting the Ground Rules

When taking the history from more than 1 person (eg, a patient, spouse and/or adult children), the patient and family members should be seated next to each other, not across from one another. The physician should be able to see the reactions of family members to the patient's answers, and responses from family members often are guarded when the patient is looking at them. Family members also may try to coax or coach the patient's responses. Not only is it easier to maintain control over the interview if the physician can see the patient and all family members at the same time, more information, often unspoken, is also gleaned.

Interviewing the Patient

The interview may be introduced by saying to the patient, "First I'd like to ask you some questions and then, if it is OK with you, I'd like to ask your [family] some questions." This request is rarely denied. It gives the patient the first chance to express concerns and promotes establishment of the doctor-patient relationship. Begin with an open-ended question to the patient, such as "Why are you here today?" If the appointment is specifically to address cognitive symptoms, the answer may reveal important information about the patient's insight. If the patient does not volunteer cognitive complaints, ask specifically "How is your memory?" "Memory" in lay terms typically covers a broad range of cognitive deficits. If deficits are acknowledged, ask the patient how long he or she has been aware of it, and if it causes problems. Ask if the patient feels clear-headed or confused, which may suggest delirium. Ask about mood and general health. Usually this entire interview with the patient is brief.

Do not let family interrupt when interviewing the patient, or let the patient defer to the family, noting, "They'll get their chance." Such interruptions or deferrals are telling, but it is also important for the physician and family to hear what the patient believes the problem to be. It may be useful to reiterate for the patient what you have heard.

Investigating the Family

With the patient's permission, which is almost invariably granted, direct further questions to the family/informant. An important first inquiry is to establish the frequency of contact the family member has with the patient. Sometimes the family member sees the patient infrequently or has reestablished ties only recently. If someone who knows the patient well did not attend the visit, find out why. Such information may not be volunteered but obviously is important.

Onset and Course

Ask of the informant, "Does [the patient] have a [cognitive] problem?" If yes, the onset and course are critical to establishing a cause. Often, family members wish to emphasize recent changes that have prompted the current evaluation. Slowing evolving changes that have caused problems in the recent past are very different from acute or subacute changes that truly began only recently. A useful question is, "When was the last time [the patient's] thinking and memory was 100%?" Disregard reported age-related changes. Patients and families, and often clinicians, may want to attribute changes to "normal aging," but such changes are rarely evident outside of a formal neuropsychological assessment. Older adults are expected to manage complex medications, finances, and social relationships. Many are fully engaged in demanding careers. Changes resulting from disease are much more often attributed incorrectly to "normal aging" than are changes of normal aging attributed incorrectly to disease.

The Major Causes of Brain Disease

The major causes of brain disease tend to have characteristic onsets and courses: vascular events (stroke) and head trauma are acute; infectious/inflammatory conditions are subacute, usually evolving over hours to days and, rarely, weeks; neoplasms are subacute, but typically evolve over weeks to months; toxic/metabolic conditions are usually subacute, also over weeks to months, and fluctuate with the underlying cause; and degenerative brain disease has an indolent but inexorably progressive course, with symptoms typically apparent for a year or more before an evaluation. Because families often report changes as sudden, a useful question is, "Have you ever thought he/she was having a stroke?"

Neurodegenerative Diseases

Neurodegenerative diseases, primarily Alzheimer disease (AD),[3] but also diffuse Lewy body disease (LBD)[4] and frontotemporal dementias (FTDs),[5] are the major causes of cognitive disorders in older adults (**Box 1**). If symptoms are progressive but only gradually so, the longer ago they began, the more likely the primary underlying etiology is neurodegenerative. When the onset is ambiguous but claimed to be recent, look for evidence that symptoms were present further back in time. Clues include mistakes in the patient's management of his or her job, finances, medications, or other instrumental activities of daily living (IADLs; ie, the ADLs beyond basic self-care that are needed to function independently). The further back in time the symptoms began, the more likely the origin is neurodegenerative disease.

Nature of Symptoms

The nature of symptoms provides other important clues to the etiology of cognitive impairment, and directed questions may be most useful for this purpose (**Box 2**).

Box 1
Common dementias and their frequency[a]

1. Alzheimer disease (60%–80%)

2. Diffuse Lewy body disease (5%–10%)

   a. Dementia with Lewy bodies

   b. Parkinson disease dementia

   c. Multiple system atrophy

3. Frontotemporal dementia (FTD) (12%–25%)[b]

   a. Behavioral variant

   b. Language variant

      i. Primary progressive aphasia—expressive aphasia

      ii. Semantic dementia—receptive aphasia

   c. Motor variant

      i. Progressive supranuclear palsy

      ii. Corticobasal degeneration

      iii. FTD with parkinsonism

      iv. FTD with amyotrophic lateral sclerosis

4. Vascular dementia (10%–20%)[c]

5. Mixed etiology (10%–30%)

  [a] Overlapping abnormalities are common.
  [b] Most FTD is young onset, <65 years old.
  [c] Vascular dementia is not consistently defined. In the absence of significant strokes involving gray matter, the contribution of cerebrovascular disease to cognitive impairment is speculative.
  Data from Refs.[3,19,20]

Box 2
The history

- Set the ground rules
  - Patient and family members next to—not across from—each other
  - Begin with patient but keep it brief. Do not allow family to interrupt
  - With the patient's permission, direct questions primarily to family
  - Patient should be present throughout
- Define onset and course or cognitive symptoms
  - When was the patient last completely normal?
    - Disregard "normal aging"
    - Onset is not when "things got bad"
  - Have symptoms progressed and, if so, gradually or suddenly?
    - Have you ever thought the patient was having a stroke?
- Define nature of cognitive symptoms
  - Memory:
    - Repeating?
    - Misplacing?
    - Relying more on notes/calendars?
    - Forgetting names of familiar persons?
  - Language:
    - Trouble finding words?
  - Visuospatial/executive function:
    - Lost driving or other driving issues?
    - Mistakes with medications or finances?
    - Difficulty with former skills?
      - Preparing a meal
      - Household repairs
      - Using tools/appliances
    - Safety concerns?
- Address associated behavior changes
  - Depressed, anxious, agitated?
  - Personality change?
    - Impulsive, inappropriate
    - Loss of empathy
  - Visual hallucination?
  - Paranoia?
  - Sleep disruption?
  - Involuntary movements or gait disturbance?

Families and mildly impaired patients typically recognize symptoms with little or no explanation from the examiner. Does he or she misplace? Struggle with names of familiar persons? Rely more on notes and calendars? [typically reflecting memory deficits] Get lost driving? [memory or visuospatial deficits] Have trouble finding words? [language deficits] Of course, all of these symptoms must reflect a decline from an earlier baseline.

Patients are rarely aware of repeating themselves (a typical symptom even early in the course of AD), but families typically readily recognize the simple question, "Does he/she repeat?" Frequent repetition of questions, often verbatim by the patient, can be exasperating for families.

Inquiries directed at executive functioning can be challenging. Executive functions refer to skills typically localized to the frontal lobes and involve organizing, planning, execution, and judgment. The ability to sequence, shift sets, and multi-task are all dependent on executive functions, and deficits may cause difficulty preparing a meal, completing a household repair, or preparing financial documents. Perhaps fortunately, executive dysfunction is often misinterpreted as a memory problem, because patients appear to have forgotten how to do things. Executive deficits are common in dementia, including AD, and are the hallmark of FTDs. A simple question that may encompass executive dysfunction is, "Do you have safety concerns [for the patient]?"

Remarkably, despite the ready endorsement by families of many or all of the cognitive deficits described, it is often a surprise to them that the patient may have trouble managing medications or finances. Even more remarkable, patients who are acknowledged to be dependent on others for virtually all IADLs, and even those needing assistance with basic ADLs, are thought by family to be safe drivers. Often, no family members have ridden with or observed the patient's driving.

Although it is important to return to driving or to other issues that relate directly to the patient's independence, do not let these matters sidetrack the evaluation.

Investigating Behavioral Symptoms

Behavioral changes are universal in brain disorders that cause cognitive impairment.[6] Asking the family about the patient's mood is important, but one must be aware that vegetative signs reflecting apathy, not depression, may accompany even early symptoms of dementia. It may take a skilled geropsychiatrist to differentiate the apathy of dementia from true depression that often accompanies dementia.[7] Older adults with cognitive disorders may improve significantly with treatment of their comorbid mood disorder, but depression, anxiety, mania, and other psychiatric conditions rarely develop as a primary disorder in late life. Even in the absence of overt cognitive impairment, such patients should be watched for an evolving neurodegenerative disorder.

Personality Change

Many changes in behavior may be interpreted as a personality change, but true personality change, characterized by impulsive, odd, and inappropriate behavior, apathy and indifference, or coarsening of affect with loss of empathy are hallmarks of behavioral variant FTD and also can be seen in traumatic brain injury (TBI). Such patients may appear quite normal in the clinic and may test well on structured mental-status examinations. Often, only the people who know them best recognize the change. When the patient appears normal and the family appears distressed, think frontal lobes.

Hallucinations and Delusions

Visual hallucinations are relatively specific to LBD (synucleinopathies),[8] particularly early in the disease course, and should be asked about in all older adults with suspected cognitive impairment. Auditory hallucinations are much less specific and are not common in the early course of dementia. Delusions, which are common in dementia, may be reported by the family as hallucinations based on the patient's statements of having seen or heard things. Confirm that family members have observed the patient hallucinating and are not just reporting what the patient has said.

Patients may be more prone to misinterpret sights or sounds (illusions), sometimes attributing a threatening quality to them. Forgetfulness and impaired judgment also can trigger paranoid delusions and may prompt accusations of stealing or other bad behavior. Pleasant delusions, such as the patient believing he or she recently visited with a long-dead friend, also may occur and, while sometimes upsetting to families, are not harmful and may actually offer opportunities to engage the patient in conversation.

Sleep

Sleep changes are common in older adults, and disrupted sleep can exacerbate cognitive symptoms. However, it is uncommon for sleep disorders to be the primary cause of cognitive impairment. The treatment of sleep apnea, restless legs, or other disorders causing excessive daytime sleepiness can improve attention but rarely eliminates the perceived changes in cognitive impairment. Rapid eye movement behavior disturbance, a sleep disorder characterized by often dramatic motor activity accompanying vivid dreams, is suggestive of LBD,[9] as are visual hallucinations.

Motor Disturbances

Involuntary movements and/or a gait disturbance may suggest LBD, a motor variant FTD, or, in another context, a toxic encephalopathy (delirium). Lateralized weakness or numbness may suggest focal brain lesions, such as stroke, subdural hematoma, or TBI. Bowel or bladder disturbance or symptoms of presyncope may indicate dysautonomia, also seen in LBD (multiple system atrophy).

The Past Medical History

A complete medical history is important, with particular emphasis on prior neurologic or psychiatric problems. In general, the brain is a resilient organ which, given enough time, can compensate for significant impairment to other organs. Apart from end-stage pulmonary, cardiac, hepatic, or renal disease, patients have at least intermittent mental clarity.

Medications

A review of medications with special attention to adherence and to drugs with central nervous system activity, including over-the-counter and illicit drugs, is important. Stable doses over years of benzodiazepines, opiates, antiepileptic drugs, or even alcohol are not likely to present as a progressive cognitive impairment unless blood levels are increasing and/or tolerance is decreasing. Not infrequently, patients with cognitive impairment make medication errors. In addition, common behavioral and psychological symptoms of dementia may lead to self-medication with drugs or alcohol.

The Family History

The family history is important, particularly if there is a strong history of mid-life neurodegenerative disease. The vast majority of dementia is sporadic, and late-life dementia in a relative condones only a mild increase in risk. Nevertheless, it is often a concern that prompts the patient to seek an evaluation.

The Social History

The patient's education, occupation, current activities and hobbies, home life, social support, and belief systems are all important factors that influence the presentation of cognitive symptoms.

The Review of Systems

Though often mandatory, the review of systems from an unreliable historian is virtually worthless. A standard form that the patient can review with a knowledgable family member before the visit to the clinic is preferred.

Interviewing the Family Separately

Although families often want to speak to the physician independently, it is best to address issues of cognitive impairment as openly and honestly as possible with the patient present. Beyond the ethical issues, deceiving or withholding information from the patient may sabotage the doctor-patient relationship. Patients may be forgetful, but they usually recognize whom they trust. Moreover, when families are reluctant to speak in front of the patient, the patient typically has limited insight and fairly significant cognitive impairment. In such situations, families are usually unduly concerned about what the patient will remember. The patient often is indifferent or, if upset, has a short-lived irritation. For patients who are more mildly or even questionably impaired, there is rarely justification for discussing concerns with the family without the patient being present.

The process of diagnosing dementia may be stressful for patients, families, and physicians, but trying to spare patients from potentially bad news is a poor strategy for managing any disease. Usually, when the physician is straightforward families do not feel the need to speak apart from the patient, and both patient and family are grateful for the physician's honesty.

THE EXAMINATION
Background

Although a general medical examination is important, the neurologic examination is key to diagnosing cognitive impairment. Observations about the patient's psychological state, including mood, affect, character of speech, thought content, and insight may influence the assessment, but in the cooperative and attentive older adult, cognitive impairment usually can be detected unless psychiatric symptoms are extreme.

The Neurologic Examination

The neurologic examination uses a carefully constructed approach to localize lesions within the nervous system. Findings are addressed in a deliberate fashion, beginning at one end of the neural axis (brain cortex) and sequentially adding considerations of other nervous system components. The mental status, reflecting function of the cerebral hemispheres, is considered first. The cranial nerves add a consideration of the brainstem. The motor examination adds the spinal cord, efferent nerves, neuromuscular junction, and muscle. The sensory examination adds afferent nerves and ascending spinal cord pathways that eventually relay in the thalamus and project to cortex. Lastly, coordination, station, and gait testing adds a consideration of cerebellar and basal ganglia input, which work through the motor system and depend on sensory feedback.

Localizing Cognitive Functions

In the alert (eyes open) and attentive (maintains eye contact) adult, the major spheres of cognition are memory, language, and visuospatial and executive function (**Fig. 1**). Each localizes to important brain regions.

The critical structures for making new memories are the hippocampi, deep in the medial temporal lobes. Language localizes to the dominant (usually left) temporoparietal cortex, visuospatial function to a similar region of the nondominant hemisphere, and executive function to the frontal lobes (**Fig. 2**). Note that language, visuospatial function, and executive function are neocortically based, whereas memory depends on the much more primitive archicortex of the hippocampus. Neorcortical deficits may be difficult to identify in the clinic, particularly in a well-educated patient. Recent or "short-term" memory, the crucial ability to learn and remember new information, tends to be easier to test and is usually affected first and foremost in AD.

Orientation is not useful for localization, is not sensitive to cognitive dysfunction, and has no uniformly recognized criteria. If a patient presents at the correct time and place, little is gained by quizzing orientation.

The Mental-Status Examination

The initial mental-status examination should be administered in a rigorous fashion, ideally by a nurse or other support staff trained in the administration of standard tests. Many such tests are available.[10,11] If there is no reason to expect cognitive dysfunction, a brief (~2 minutes) screen, such as the Mini-Cog™,[12] is adequate. If problems are suspected, a more extensive test, such as the Montreal Cognitive Assessment

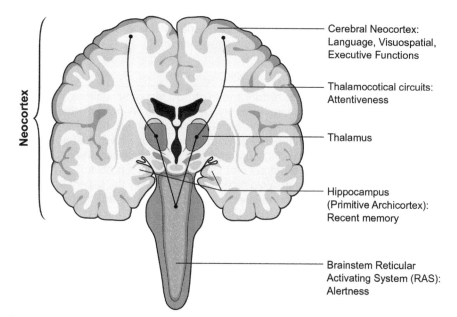

Fig. 1. Structures that are midline and deeper in the brain are more primitive. After recovery from an acute, bilateral insult to the brain (eg, anoxia), alertness requires only the reticular activating system. Attentiveness requires thalamic drivers to keep the cortex in a receptive state. Recent or "short-term" memory is dependent on the hippocampi, a primitive archicortex. Language, visuospatial, and executive functions are all more evolved, depend on the neocortex, and may be difficult to assess in a brief examination.

Neocortex

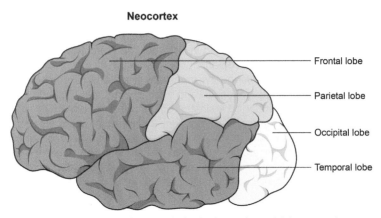

Frontal lobe

Parietal lobe

Occipital lobe

Temporal lobe

Fig. 2. Neocortical structures, and particularly the large frontal lobes, are the most evolved and dynamic part of the brain. Only about 10% of neocortex is primary sensory (vision, hearing, touch, smell, taste) or motor (output) cortex. The vast areas of association cortex create the individual's perception of the world, act on those perceptions, and otherwise "think." Though critical to the individual's function, they may be challenging to test in the clinic.

(MoCA),[13] can be used. The scores on such tests are not diagnostic but do alert the physician to the potential need for further evaluation.

It is essential for the physician have a good working knowledge of cognitive function to help decide if (1) the patient is a reliable historian and responsible partner in recommended cares; and (2) further testing is needed and, if so, what.

Families should be invited to observe the mental-status examination. Not infrequently, they are shocked at the patient's performance.

Recent Memory

Because of its importance to the history and treatment recommendations, it is imperative that the recent or short-term memory be assessed. A patient with impaired recent memory is, de facto, an unreliable historian and also should not be accountable for adhering to treatment recommendations, including medications. Just as with any other abnormal examination finding, the physician should reassess recent memory as needed until he or she is convinced that there is or is not a problem.

Recent memory is tested by delayed recall. Most commonly the patient is asked to remember 3 unrelated words and to later recall the words after an interference (distracter) task. Not all words lists are equal,[14] and a standard list, such as "leader, season, table" should be used. The interference task, not the time delay, is key to identifying deficits in recent memory and must be adequately demanding to fully engage the patient. Common interference tasks include serial 7 subtractions ("Count backwards from 100 by 7s") and reciting the months of the year in reverse order, either of which is also a good test of attention/concentration. The clock draw task, the interference task used in the Mini-Cog™, assesses visuospatial and executive function (see later discussion).

If a patient struggles to recall the 3 words after the first interference task, have the patient repeat them again, do another interference task, and again test recall. Struggling a second time is concerning. Struggling a third time, again rehearsing the words and using a different interference task, is very likely not normal. The test can be refined by providing letter or category cues, then multiple choice if needed. Patients who do not recall the words but readily get them with a simple cue (eg, "Starts with the letter," "A piece of furniture") may be intact, particularly if they later recall the words without cues. Patients who cannot recognize the words from a multiple-choice list (eg, "sugar, sailor, or season," or "chair, table, or sofa") are most concerning, particularly on repeated testing.

Well-educated patients may be able to bear down enough to appear intact on a simple quiz, but deficits may be revealed on their knowledge of current events. Major recent events, such as elections and natural catastrophes, or historic events, such as 9/11, should be recalled by anyone who acknowledges following the news. Mistakes, particularly when unrecognized by the patient, may be startling.

Language

Even when word-finding difficulties are reported, they may not be apparent when talking with the patient. Asking the patient to follow multiple step instructions—essentially, 3-stage commands—is a simple test of comprehension and can be incorporated into most examinations. Be deliberate in giving the patient multiple instructions at once, without cues, as opposed to a series of 1-step instructions. For example, say, "Hold your hands straight out in front of you, elbows straight, palms up, at shoulder level, and close your eyes" [instructions for testing drift]. Decide what is important for any routine examination and invent a way to incorporate a multistage command into that examination. This approach represents an efficient use of time and reveals something of the patient's likelihood of being able to follow advice.

Generative Naming

Generative naming may be revealing, even when conversation and comprehension appear intact. Semantic (category) fluency tends to reflect temporal lobe functions, whereas phonemic (letter) fluency taps into frontal lobe function.[15] Patients are given 1 minute to generate as many names, typically animals, or words beginning with a specific letter, typically f, a, or s. Jot down the starting time to the second, as tracking words can be demanding. Normally patients generate at least 11 words per minute. Patients with AD may have more difficulty with categories, whereas FTD patients may have trouble with letters.

Naming objects is difficult to qualify and quantify in the clinic, and may be intact until deficits are relatively severe. It is also less revealing than difficulties following instructions or generating words.

Be aware that intact language skills do not preclude significant deficits in memory, visuospatial function, or executive function. Often, even severely cognitively impaired patients appear normal because of preserved language and social skills, basically "talking a good game," and fooling both family and providers.

Visuospatial Skills

Visuospatial skills are difficult to test in the clinic, despite the profound impact such deficits may have on function. Their assessment often overlaps with that of executive function. Copying intersecting pentagons, in which 2 5-sided figures form a 4-sided intersection, or copying a cube such that the figure appears 3-dimensional, the appropriate lines are parallel and of equal length, and no lines are added, are relatively specific bedside tests for visuospatial deficits.

Executive Function

Executive functions are the most evolved and complex of biological functions in the known universe. Almost half of the brain—the frontal lobes—is dedicated to executive functions. These functions also may be most important to successful independent living, because they are the basis of planning, organizing, recognizing patterns, shifting attention as needed, and making sound judgments. Nevertheless, deficits may be difficult to recognize in the clinic. Because they are so involved in interpersonal interactions, it is not surprising that persons who know the patient best may recognize changes before others. Facial expression, body language, and tone of voice may speak volumes to family members but mean little to a relative stranger.

It must be reiterated here that when a patient appears normal and has no complaints, but the family looks distressed, think frontal lobes.

The Clock-Draw Task

The clock-draw task taps into both visuospatial and executive functions (planning, abstracting), and is an efficient way to screen for either. There are a variety of ways to score the clock. Basically all 12 numbers should be present, in order, only once, in the correct clockwise direction, and the hands should point to the correct numbers. Ideally the drawing should be well planned, with quadrants defined, numbers correctly spaced, and hands of the appropriate length. The time "11:10" is most often used, the instruction being, "Place the hands at 11:10, 10 minutes past 11." Impaired patients are often "stimulus bound," and tend to draw hands pointing to the 10 and 11. Other times, including 8:20 and 1:45, also require abstraction and are only slightly less likely to reveal deficits.[14]

Sequencing

Sequencing may be challenging for patients with executive dysfunctions, if not more global cognitive impairment.[16] The Luria sequencing task, or fist-edge-palm test, is administered as follows. Instruct the patient to "Watch me." Do not provide any verbal cues. Demonstrate the sequence of fist (fingers balled, perpendicular to the floor), edge (hand open, perpendicular to the floor), palm (hand open, parallel to floor), tapping your hand on your thigh as you perform each movement. Use a silent 4-count beat (1 beat rest after each sequence) to clearly distinguish the 3 steps. Perform the demonstration 3 times, and then say to the patient, "Now you do it." A normal patient performs this readily, 3 times in a row. If the patient does not perform it correctly 3 times, say "Do it with me," and demonstrate 3 more trials, making sure the patient mimics your hand position. Then say "Keep going." The test is scored as spontaneously correct, correct with coaching, partially correct (1 or 2, but not 3 correct sequences in a row), or unable to do.

Set-Shifting

Set-shifting is another challenging task for persons with frontal lobe dysfunction, and also for those with any significant deficits in attention (delirium). Trails B is a neuropsychological test whereby numbers and letters are randomly distributed on a page and the patient must connect them in the correct, alternating sequence: 1-A-2-B-3-C, and so forth.

Trails B can be administered orally, tapping into executive function, attention, and working memory. Say to the patient, "Complete this sequence: 1-A-2-B-3-C." Most can complete the entire sequence, arriving at 26-Z or close to it. Those with executive dysfunction often charge ahead but quickly lose track of the sequence, responding incorrectly with all numbers or letters, or sequences that are clearly out of order. Those with even subtle delirium, (eg, mild intoxication or medication side effects) may quickly lose their place. Patients able to complete this task are unlikely to have delirium, and any other cognitive deficits identified are usually the product of brain disease.

The oral Trails B task is also an excellent interference task for testing memory. It is virtually impossible to rehearse newly presented information, thereby enhancing delayed recall, and correctly attend to this task.

As noted under language function, phonemic fluency (the number of words generated in 1 minute beginning with f, a, or s) also tends to be disproportionately impaired in disorders affecting the frontal lobes.

Other clinical assessments of executive/frontal lobe function often have biases and are difficult to quantify, but can be revealing to the experienced clinician. The interpretation of proverbs depends on the patient's age, culture, and education. The response demonstrating the optimal abstraction is another proverb of the same meaning. Interpreting similarities and differences (eg, how are an orange and a banana alike?) may be complicated by creative responses (both are good sources of potassium).

The Remainder of the Neurologic Examination

The neurologic examination is often seen as overly complex and time consuming, but most findings relevant to the differential diagnosis of cognitive impairment can be gathered in short order (**Box 3**).

It is much better to make a few valid, reproducible observations than to make generalizations such as "grossly intact," "nonfocal," or "nonlateralizing." Each of the following descriptions of a normal examination take only moments to observe or test, yet are of high yield in terms of assessing the integrity of the nervous system outside of the mental status.

Cranial nerves: Visual fields full, extraocular movements (EOMs) intact, face symmetric, speech articulate, hearing intact to soft voice.

Stands easily from a chair without pushing off, gait normal, walks well on tiptoes and heels, station normal, postural reflexes intact, Romberg negative, Drift negative, finger-to-nose testing and rapid alternating movements intact.

In the most abbreviated neurologic examination, apart from always testing recent memory, the EOMs and the gait are the most important to test. Develop skill in watching for smooth, seamless pursuit movements without evidence of intrusion saccades. The observation of a normal gait, which is readily recognized, may be an invaluable piece of information to document and track.

ADDITIONAL TESTING
Brain Imaging

Frequently, brain imaging (magnetic resonance imaging or computed tomography) is used as a substitute for the neurologic examination. The brain is tremendously dynamic, and a static picture may reveal little about neurologic function. The most common cognitive disorders, namely neurodegenerative dementias, are not evident on routine imaging, and functional imaging is confirmatory at best, not diagnostic. The strongest argument for brain imaging for cognitive impairment is that the patient is typically an unreliable historian, and a significant injury or event may be forgotten. Many "abnormal" findings on imaging are nonspecific (eg, the ubiquitous "small-vessel ischemic disease," which may or may not represent vascular disease) and of no clinical significance. Imaging does rule out significant cortical strokes, TBIs, tumors, subdural hematomas, and hydrocephalus, any of which could cause or aggravate cognitive symptoms.

Laboratory

Vitamin B_{12} and thyroid-stimulating hormone are the only laboratory tests that commonly are not already part of the clinical laboratory data. A complete blood count,

Box 3
High-yield neurologic examination findings in the evaluation of cognitive symptoms

Cranial Nerves

- Extraocular movements (cranial nerves III, IV, VI)
  - Rationale: Assesses the most discrete of motor movements, requiring multiple coordinated areas of brain function. Abnormal in:
    - Progressive supranuclear palsy, Parkinson disease
    - Some structural lesions
    - Drug toxicity
    - All brain disease, at least subtly
  - Procedure: "Follow my finger with your eyes"
    - Move finger to extremes of gaze at varying speeds
    - Observe particularly for smoothness of pursuit movements
    - Do not hold finger too close, as difficulty converging (older adults) may produce nonpathologic intrusion saccades (choppy eye movements)
  - Normal: Seamless, conjugate pursuit of target
  - Abnormal:
    - Dysconjugate or lack of full range of motion (± mildly limited up gaze in older adults)
    - Significant nystagmus (beyond mild, symmetric end point)
    - Decrease in smoothness of pursuit movements (nonspecific but sensitive)
- Speech (cranial nerves V, VII, IX, X, XII)
  - Rationale: Multiple brain and peripheral structures are involved. May be abnormal in:
    - Bilateral corticobulbar (pseudobulbar) lesions
    - Bulbar (lower brainstem) lesions
    - Basal ganglia and cerebellar disorders
    - Some lateralized structural lesions
    - Drug toxicity
  - Procedure: Assess speech quality during interview
  - Normal: Speech articulate, volume normal
  - Abnormal:
    - Dysarthria (slurred; eg, cerebellar/brainstem lesions, drug toxicity)
    - Hypophonia (eg, Parkinson disease)
    - Halting (eg, basal ganglia, language cortex)
    - Dysphonia (hoarseness)/nasal speech (brainstem or peripheral structures)

Drift

- *Rationale*: May detect lateralized motor, sensory, cerebellar deficits; highly reproducible
- *Procedure*: Arms extended, palms up, shoulder level, eyes closed
- *Normal*: Holds for 10 seconds; tremor is discounted
- *Abnormal*: One arm
  - Pronates, may also drift downward (corticospinal tract lesion)
  - Drifts laterally to 45° (ipsilateral cerebellar dysfunction)
  - Drifts upward (may be central sensory deficit)

Stand

- *Rationale*: Detects weakness, postural instability that poses risk of falls; highly reproducible
- *Procedure*: Cross arms over chest and stand up
- *Normal*: Patient stands easily without pushing off
- *Abnormal*:
  - Struggles but stands without pushing off
  - Must push off to stand
  - Needs assistance to stand
  - Cannot stand

Gait

- *Rationale*: Requires integrated motor, sensory, basal ganglia, cerebellar function. Gait is often abnormal in:
  - Lewy body disease
    - Untreated Parkinson disease
    - Dementia with Lewy bodies
    - Multiple system atrophy
  - Tau disorders
    - Progressive supranuclear palsy
    - Corticobasal degeneration
    - Other frontotemporal dementias
  - Huntington disease
  - Post–cardiovascular accident or traumatic brain injury
  - Normal pressure hydrocephalus
  - Cerebellar or toxic/metabolic disorders
- Procedure: Tell patient, "Take a fast walk down the hall [to bring out abnormalities]." Then, "Come on back [to observe turns]." Note:
  - Base
  - Stride
  - Posture
  - Arm swing
  - Turns
- Normal: Walks normally 30 ft down the hallway and returns
- Abnormal:
  - Hemiplegic/paretic (lateralized brain lesion)
  - Parkinsonian (basal ganglia, relative dopamine deficiency)
  - Choreiform (basal ganglia, relative dopamine excess)
  - Ataxic (cerebellar; alcohol intoxication causes classic gait ataxia)
  - Magnetic/apractic (normal pressure hydrocephalus and frontal lobe disorders)
  - Neuropathic (peripheral nerve; steppage gait in extreme cases)
  - Myopathic (muscle; may cause waddling with weakness of pelvic girdle)
  - Antalgic (nonneurologic gait disturbance related to pain)

liver and renal function tests, glucose, electrolytes, and calcium should be documented. When appropriate, testing should be done for sexually transmitted disease (rapid plasma reagin, human immunodeficiency virus). The onset, course, and nature of symptoms may dictate further evaluations (eg, Lyme titers, drug and heavy metal screens) but are infrequently indicated and should not be pursued in what appears to be a typical case of AD, LBD, or FTD.

Neuropsychological Testing

Formal neuropsychological testing is invaluable when assessing truly mild or questionable symptoms of cognitive impairment. Each of the major domains of cognition already outlined is assessed with multiple, standardized tests. The neuropsychologist with an interest in older adults may be skilled at diagnosing AD versus LBD versus FTD. Not all neuropsychologists have the same skill sets, and some are much less willing than others to endorse a pattern suggesting an irreversible, progressive brain disease. The neuropsychologist may place undue weight on the report of neuroimaging (small-vessel ischemic disease), vascular risk factors, and a history of alcohol use.

Functional Assessments

Occupational therapists may be skilled at assessing ADLs and IADLs in older adults. A structured, performance-based evaluation, such as the Cognitive Performance Test,[17] has the advantage of allowing family members to observe as patients are directed to perform various tasks. Prompts are provided in a graded fashion until the task is completed, revealing the degree of assistance needed. Such information may be crucial in deciding if the patient has the "impairment in function" that is integral to the definition of dementia, and can be telling about the safety of the patient's current activities and environment.

Other Tests

When indicated, a sleep study should be pursued before neuropsychological testing. An electroencephalogram occasionally is helpful if there is a true question of spells of confusion, or if a subacute progression suggestive of prion disease is suspected.

It is important to recognize that the vast majority of cognitive disorders are clinical diagnoses, and ancillary tests rarely identify a reversible cause.[18]

THE ASSESSMENT

The physician's first job is to decide if there is: (1) no cognitive impairment; (2) cognitive impairment, not dementia; or (3) dementia. For either of the latter 2 possibilities a specific etiology should be sought, which will directly relate to the prognosis and steer the patient and family to the resources needed.

REFERENCES

1. Valcour VG, Masaki KH, Curb JD, et al. The detection of dementia in the primary care setting. Arch Intern Med 2000;160:2964–8.
2. Chodosh J, Petitti DB, Elliott M, et al. Physician recognition of cognitive impairment: evaluating the need for improvement. J Am Geriatr Soc 2004;52:1051–9.
3. Plassman BL, Langa KM, Fisher GG, et al. Prevalence of dementia in the United States: the aging, demographics, and memory study. Neuroepidemiology 2007; 29:125–32.

4. Schneider JA, Arvanitakis Z, Yu L, et al. Cognitive impairment, decline and fluc-tuations in older community-dwelling subjects with Lewy bodies. Brain 2012;135: 3005–14.

5. Baborie A, Griffiths TD, Jaros E, et al. Pathological correlates of frontotemporal lobar degeneration in the elderly. Acta Neuropathol 2011;121:365–71.

6. Casanova MF, Starkstein SE, Jellinger KA. Clinicopathological correlates of behavioral and psychological symptoms of dementia. Acta Neuropathol 2011; 122:117–35.

7. Wright SL, Persad C. Distinguishing between depression and dementia in older persons: neuropsychological and neuropathological correlates. J Geriatr Psychi-atry Neurol 2007;20:189–98.

8. Burghaus L, Eggers C, Timmermann L, et al. Hallucinations in neurodegenerative diseases. CNS Neurosci Ther 2012;18:149–59.

9. Zanigni S, Calandra-Buonaura G, Grimaldi D, et al. REM behaviour disorder and neurodegenerative diseases. Sleep Med 2011;12(Suppl 2):S54–8.

10. Ashford JW. Screening for memory disorders, dementia and Alzheimer's disease. Aging Health 2008;4:399–432.

11. Brodaty H, Low LF, Gibson L, et al. What is the best dementia screening instru-ment for general practitioners to use? Am J Geriatr Psychiatry 2006;14:391–400.

12. Borson S, Scanlan JM, Chen P, et al. The Mini-Cog as a screen for dementia: vali-dation in a population-based sample. J Am Geriatr Soc 2003;51:1451–4.

13. Nasreddine ZS, Phillips NA, Bedirian V, et al. The Montreal cognitive assessment, MoCA: a brief screening tool for mild cognitive impairment. J Am Geriatr Soc 2005;53:695–9.

14. McCarten JR, Anderson P, Kuskowski MA, et al. Screening for cognitive impair-ment in an elderly veteran population: acceptability and results using different versions of the Mini-Cog. J Am Geriatr Soc 2011;59:309–13.

15. Tupak SV, Badewien M, Dresler T, et al. Differential prefrontal and frontotemporal oxygenation patterns during phonemic and semantic verbal fluency. Neuropsy-chologia 2012;50:1565–9.

16. Weiner MF, Hynan LS, Rossetti H, et al. Luria's three-step test: what is it and what does it tell us? Int Psychogeriatr 2011;23:1602–6.

17. Burns T, Mortimer JA, Merchak P. Cognitive performance test: a new approach to functional assessment in Alzheimer's disease. J Geriatr Psychiatry Neurol 1994;7: 46–54.

18. Clarfield AM. The decreasing prevalence of reversible dementias: an updated meta-analysis. Arch Intern Med 2003;163:2219–29.

19. Holsinger T, Deveau J, Boustani M, et al. Does this patient have dementia? JAMA 2007;297:2391–404.

20. Daviglus ML, Bell CC, Berrettini W, et al. NIH state-of-the-science conference statement: preventing Alzheimer's disease and cognitive decline. NIH Consens State Sci Statements 2010;27:1–30.

Emerging Biomarkers in Cognition

Meredith Wicklund, MD[a], Ronald C. Petersen, MD, PhD[b],*

KEYWORDS

- Biomarkers • Dementia • Alzheimer disease

KEY POINTS

- Biomarkers are measurable, in vivo indicators of a specific disease-related pathologic process.
- The goal of biomarkers is to provide direct evidence of an underlying pathologic process, provide indirect evidence of a pathologic process through evidence of synapse dysfunction and neurodegeneration, or provide evidence of an alternative pathologic process.
- Amyloid imaging and cerebrospinal fluid (CSF) amyloid β_{42} ($A\beta_{42}$) provide direct evidence of amyloid disorders in Alzheimer disease (AD).
- Structural magnetic resonance imaging (MRI), fluorodeoxyglucose positron emission tomography, single-photon emission computed tomography, and CSF tau can provide indirect evidence of AD as markers of synapse dysfunction and neurodegeneration, whereas certain patterns may suggest pathologic processes other than AD.
- The best CSF marker to predict conversion from mild cognitive impairment (MCI) to dementia is an abnormal ratio of $A\beta_{42}$ to total tau or abnormal levels of both markers.
- Biomarkers evolve over time and do not become abnormal or maxima at the same time but vary with the stages of the pathophysiologic process.
- Biomarker data can be applied to MCI criteria to improve diagnostic certainty that the underlying pathologic process is caused by AD.
- Several new biomarkers are in development but have not yet been approved for clinical practice, including plasma $A\beta$, markers of oxidative stress and inflammation, lipidomics, spectroscopy, functional MRI, diffusion tensor imaging, and magnetic resonance perfusion.

Disclosures: Dr M. Wicklund, none. Dr R.C. Petersen, Pfizer, Inc; Janssen Alzheimer Immunotherapy; Chair, Data Monitoring Board, Elan Pharmaceuticals; consultant, GE Healthcare; consultant and CME lecture, Novartis Inc.

[a] Division of Behavioral Neurology, Department of Neurology, Mayo Clinic, 200 1st Street Southwest, Rochester, MN 55905, USA; [b] Division of Behavioral Neurology, Department of Neurology, Mayo Alzheimer's Disease Research Center, Mayo Clinic, 200 1st Street Southwest, Rochester, MN 55905, USA
* Corresponding author.
E-mail address: peter8@mayo.edu

INTRODUCTION

Degenerative cognitive disorders, such as Alzheimer disease (AD), exist along a spectrum from a preclinical stage of individuals without symptoms but with biological predisposition[1-3] to mild cognitive impairment (MCI), being the earliest manifestation of clinical symptoms, and dementia, being the most advanced stage. The study of aging and dementia is moving toward an earlier identification of those presymptomatic and initially symptomatic individuals[4] with the goal of intervening with disease-modifying treatments. Although 40% to 60% of individuals with MCI progress to dementia over 5 years,[5,6] MCI is a heterogenous group of variable causes, some of which are treatable or reversible.[7,8] To that end, there has been considerable research in identifying markers of the underlying pathophysiologic process in those earliest stages and, recently, biomarker data have been incorporated in the updated research diagnostic criteria of MCI caused by AD.[9]

Biomarkers are measurable, in vivo indicators of a specific disease-related pathologic process. The most common underlying pathologic process in MCI is AD; thus, most of the research in biomarkers for MCI has focused on that process and is discussed in this article. The use of biomarkers in identifying AD has the following goals:[9]

1. Provide direct evidence of an underlying AD-related pathologic process
2. Provide indirect evidence of AD disorders through markers of synapse dysfunction and neurodegeneration
3. Assist in determining the stage or rate of disease progression
4. Provide evidence of alternative non-AD pathologic processes

Examples of biomarkers for each category as they relate to MCI caused by AD are provided in **Table 1**. Imaging and CSF measurements are the most widely used biomarkers. Amyloid plaques are the hallmark pathologic process in AD and amyloid positron emission tomography (PET) imaging or CSF measurement of amyloid β_{42} ($A\beta_{42}$) provide direct evidence of that process. Although tau deposition in the form of neurofibrillary tangles is also critical for the pathologic diagnosis of AD,[10] tau levels are less specific than $A\beta$ markers and may better reflect neuronal injury and synapse loss; thus, tau is a better indicator of neurodegeneration. Other measures of neurodegeneration include structural and functional imaging studies, namely magnetic resonance (MR)

Table 1 Biomarkers in MCI caused by AD	
Purpose	**Biomarker**
Marker of amyloid disorders in AD	PET amyloid imaging CSF $A\beta_{42}$
Marker of synapse dysfunction and neurodegeneration in AD	FDG-PET or SPECT temporoparietal hypometabolism/perfusion CSF tau Structural MRI (eg, hippocampal atrophy, cortical thinning)
Marker of disease progression from MCI to dementia caused by AD	FDG-PET or SPECT temporoparietal hypometabolism/perfusion CSF tau Structural MRI (eg, hippocampal atrophy, cortical thinning)
Marker of non-AD process	Structural MRI (eg, significant infarcts/cerebrovascular disease, subdural hematomas, tumor) FDG-PET or SPECT nontemporoparietal hypometabolism SPECT with dopamine ligands

Abbreviations: CSF, cerebrospinal fluid; FDG, fluorodeoxyglucose; PET, positron emission tomography; SPECT, single-photon emission computed tomography.

imaging (MRI) brain atrophy, fluorodeoxyglucose (FDG)-PET hypometabolism, and single-photon emission computed tomography (SPECT) hypoperfusion.

BIOMARKERS OF Aβ DEPOSITION

During the pathologic process of AD, the amyloid protein forms insoluble fibrils and is deposited extracellularly. There is considerable interest in instruments that can detect and quantify this process via imaging[11] and CSF biomarkers of amyloid deposition. However, the ability of plasma amyloid levels to directly quantify brain amyloid levels has not been firmly established[12] and is discussed elsewhere.

PET Amyloid Imaging

Amyloid imaging via a PET tracer binding to fibrillar amyloid was introduced around 2004, using the carbon 11 Pittsburgh compound B (PiB).[13] The short half-life of the PiB limits the clinical application of the test and, in April 2012, the US Food and Drug Administration (FDA) approved a fluorinated tracer, (E)-4-(2-(6-(2-(2-(2-^{18}F-fluoroethoxy)ethoxy)ethoxy)pyridin-3-yl)vinyl)-N-methyl benzenamine (^{18}F-AV-45) or florbetapir, and other fluorinated tracers are in development. This tracer has a longer half-life, allowing regional manufacturing and distribution that is not available with PiB.[14] Although an amyloid PET is interpreted as either positive, indicating the presence of tracer uptake of amyloid fibrils, or negative, indicating that is lacking the typical uptake of tracer, regional information may be useful. Compared with controls, amyloid PET scans in patients with AD show widespread uptake of tracer in cortical areas, with the most prominent uptake in the frontal cortex and precuneus followed by the parietal and temporal cortices (**Fig. 1**); minimal uptake is seen in cortical areas known to be less affected in AD, such as the primary motor, sensory, and visual cortices.[15] Temporal amyloid deposition may also be independently related to memory deficits in cognitively normal elderly patients or patients with MCI.[16]

Positive amyloid imaging correlates with AD disorders at autopsy in most, but not all, cases.[11,17–19] In MCI, a positive PiB[20,21] or florbetapir[22,23] amyloid imaging scan correlates with progression to dementia caused by AD, whereas a positive PiB scan also correlates with time to progression.[24] Although these data are convincing, precise prediction models have not yet been generated. There still can be a considerable time

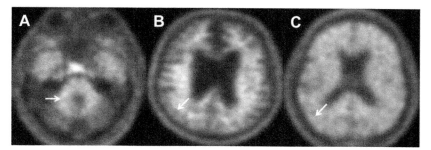

Fig. 1. Amyloid PET imaging. Axial sections of PET images obtained with the administration of ^{18}F-AV-45, or florbetapir, as a tracer for fibrillar amyloid in an individual without (*B*) and with (*C*) AD. The tracer binds nonspecifically to white matter; using cerebellar white matter as a reference (*A, arrow*), the lack of tracer uptake in cortical areas creates a distinct gray-white junction in an individual with a negative scan (*B, arrow*), whereas the gray-white junction is lost with the uptake of tracer in cortical areas in an individual with a positive scan (*C, arrow*).

lag for individuals with positive amyloid imaging scans with respect to their progression from the MCI to the dementia stage of AD, and more research needs to be done to clarify this progression pattern.

CSF Aβ₄₂

β-Amyloid protein ending at amino acid 42 (Aβ$_{42}$) is the core protein of neuritic plaques. As the protein is deposited in the brain, lower levels remain in the CSF. Low CSF Aβ$_{42}$ has been shown to correlate with pathologic diagnosis of AD at autopsy.[25,26] Across multiple studies, low CSF Aβ$_{42}$ has a mean sensitivity of greater than 85% with a specificity of 90% in detecting AD versus normal aging across studies.[27] In MCI, low CSF Aβ$_{42}$ is a predictor of progression to dementia[28–30] with similar or lower sensitivity.[27]

Because both amyloid PET imaging and CSF Aβ$_{42}$ are biomarkers of brain amyloid deposition, a positive amyloid scan should correlate with low CSF Aβ$_{42}$. This correlation has been shown,[31–34] further asserting the validity of these tests as biomarkers for amyloid deposition.

BIOMARKERS OF NEURODEGENERATION

Amyloid deposition is insufficient by itself to result in cognitive impairment. The second goal of biomarkers is therefore to provide evidence of neurodegeneration.[35] This evidence can be provided through a variety of markers, including MRI, FDG-PET, and CSF tau levels.

MRI

There has been more literature generated on the usefulness of structural MRI in predicting progression to dementia than for most of the other biomarkers.[24,36,37] Cerebral atrophy correlates with neuronal loss[38]; thus volumetric measurements on MRI, such as hippocampal atrophy, ventricular volume expansion, whole-brain atrophy, and

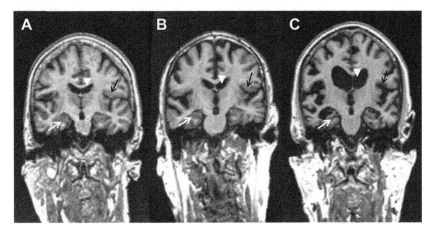

Fig. 2. MRI in cognitively normal individuals, MCI, and dementia. Coronal T1 magnetization-prepared rapid acquisition with gradient echo (MP RAGE) sections through the hippocampus in a cognitively normal individual (*A*) and individuals with MCI (*B*) and dementia caused by AD (*C*). Hippocampal atrophy (*long white arrows*), ventricular dilatation (*arrowheads*), and cortical thinning (*black arrows*) with widening of the sulci are first subtly noted in the MCI stage (*B*) and rapidly increase through the dementia stage (*C*), when they become readily apparent. These structural MRI changes are predictors of conversion from MCI to dementia.

cortical thinning can provide useful information on neurodegeneration (**Fig. 2**). Although these measurements are not specific to AD, they do predict progression from MCI to dementia.[39,40] Hippocampal atrophy can be measured both qualitatively and quantitatively. Several scales are being introduced to allow the clinician to assess medial temporal lobe atrophy in the office, and visual rating of hippocampal atrophy can be useful.[41] Automated volumetric MRI measurements have also become available through programs like FreeSurfer[42]; these are becoming more widely available for use in clinical practice, and they could soon be used in a fashion similar to bone density measures used to assess osteoporosis.[43]

FDG-PET

The brain metabolic rate directly correlates with synaptic activity.[44,45] Degenerating areas of the brain theoretically show less synaptic activity and therefore less metabolic activity. Because glucose is the fuel for the brain, a glucose-tagged PET tracer (eg, FDG) provides valuable information about the metabolic activity of the brain and thereby serves as a marker of neurodegeneration. Patients with clinical and pathologically confirmed AD show a characteristic FDG-PET pattern of hypometabolism in the bilateral temporoparietal association regions, including the posterior cingulate and precuneus, sparing the primary motor, sensory, and visual cortices,[46,47] even when correcting for cerebral atrophy (**Fig. 3**C).[48]

The temporoparietal hypometabolic pattern on FDG-PET characteristic of AD can appear before any clinical symptoms.[49] This possibility is most prominent in apolipoprotein E4 homozygotes but also has been seen in heterozygotes.[50] Among patients with MCI, the temporoparietal metabolic pattern indicates conversion to dementia (see **Fig. 3**B).[51,52]

SPECT

SPECT is an imaging technique using radioligands to measure regional cerebral blood flow (rCBF). Because brain perfusion is tightly correlated with brain metabolism, brain SPECT provides a surrogate marker similar to FDG-PET for functional brain activity, and, inversely, neurodegeneration. SPECT scans are the most widely available functional neuroimaging technologies given the relative ease of use and lower cost of the

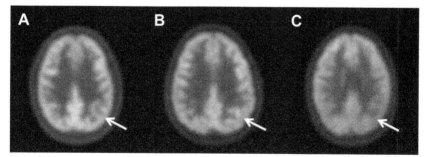

Fig. 3. FDG-PET in cognitively normal individuals, MCI, and dementia. Axial section of FDG-PET scans in a cognitively normal individual (*A*) and individuals with MCI (*B*) and dementia caused by AD (*C*). Less tracer uptake is apparent in hypometabolic areas. FDG-PET hypometabolism is a marker of neuronal injury and dysfunction. Normal tracer uptake is noted in the temporoparietal region of a cognitively normal individual (*A, white arrow*). Subtle temporoparietal hypometabolism is noted in MCI (*B, white arrow*), which is a predictor of conversion to dementia. The temporoparietal hypometabolism is more apparent in an individual with dementia caused by AD (*C, white arrow*).

radioligands compared with PET; SPECT radioligands generally have longer half-lives, do not need a cyclotron for manufacturing, and are FDA approved for brain imaging. However, PET scans have greater spatial resolution.

As with PET, SPECT scans show hypoperfusion in the posterior temporoparietal association regions sparing the primary cortices,[53] even correcting for atrophy[54] in dementia caused by AD, which correlates with neurofibrillary tangle disorders.[55] In patients with MCI, hypoperfusion in these areas predicts progression to dementia.[56,57]

Although PET and SPECT yield similar results, PET has greater spatial resolution and is less confounded by coexistent cerebrovascular disease. Direct comparisons of the 2 imaging modalities have shown greater sensitivity and overall accuracy for PET versus SPECT, even when using high-resolution SPECT scanners.[58,59]

CSF Tau

Tau protein plays a key role in the disorders of AD.[10] In AD, tau accumulates in neurons, disrupting normal activity and causing its release into the extracellular space. CSF tau levels are therefore increased in AD,[60,61] and this finding correlates with the presence of neurofibrillary tangles in the pathologic diagnosis of AD.[62,63] Likewise, normal CSF tau levels are found in AD mimickers, such as depression,[64] alcoholic dementia,[65] and Parkinson disease (PD),[66] aiding in the discrimination of these diseases.

However, increased CSF tau is not specific for AD and can be seen in a variety of neurologic conditions, such as stroke, traumatic brain injury, or prion diseases.[67–69] The intensity of increased CSF tau reflects the intensity of neurodegeneration. In AD, phosphorylated tau is the principal component of neurofibrillary tangles.[70] Because phosphotau is not increased in stroke[67] or Creutzfeldt-Jakob disease,[71] increased CSF levels of phosphotau may provide improved diagnostic discrimination from AD. Phosphotau levels may also aid in discrimination from frontotemporal dementia[72] or dementia with Lewy bodies.[73]

Total tau levels have been more extensively studied than phosphotau; there is a mean sensitivity greater than 80% to differentiate AD from nondemented aged individuals.[27] Increased levels of CSF total tau are also predictors of progression from MCI to dementia,[28–30] with similar or lower sensitivity.[27] Phosphotau levels have a similar specificity (around 80%), with modest improvement in sensitivity (to 92%) in discriminating AD from nondemented aged individuals.[27] Phosphotau can likewise predict conversion from MCI to dementia.[28,74] However, there is a large variation in these sensitivity and specificity figures across studies, and these studies examine different phosphorylated tau epitopes.[27] Likewise, there is large variability in assay results across different centers, with no standardization of analytical techniques or clinical procedures.[29]

Combinations of CSF Markers

All 3 CSF markers discussed ($A\beta_{42}$, total tau, and phosphotau), can independently predict conversion from MCI to dementia (**Table 2**). Several studies have examined

Table 2	
CSF biomarkers in MCI caused by AD	
Biomarker	**Level**
$A\beta_{42}$	Low
Total tau	High
Phosphotau	High
$A\beta_{42}$/total tau	Low

whether combinations of these markers improve diagnostic accuracy. A meta-analysis found that the best predictor of conversion is an abnormal ratio of $A\beta_{42}$ to total tau or abnormal levels of both markers; the addition of phosphotau did not have added benefit.[75] This combination of markers produces a sensitivity of 87% with a specificity of 70% and positive predictive value of 65%.[75]

BIOMARKERS OF NON-AD PROCESSES

The last role of biomarkers is to exclude other pathologic processes that may account for cognitive impairment. Any of the biomarkers discussed earlier can be helpful in this regard. Structural brain MRI can show, among other things, cerebral infarcts, significant cerebrovascular white matter disease, subdural hematomas, hydrocephalus, or tumors underlying a cognitive process. Furthermore, the posterior temporoparietal hypometabolism and hypoperfusion pattern via FDG-PET and SPECT, respectively, is distinct from that seen in other neurodegenerative disorders, such as frontotemporal lobar degeneration (FTLD) or dementia with Lewy bodies (DLB), which can appear similar clinically (**Fig. 4**); for example, hypometabolism in FTLD is most prominent in the anterior frontal and temporal lobes.[76] FDG-PET can thereby improve diagnostic accuracy between these two disorders,[77] but does not define these disorders because frontal variants of AD can appear similar.[78,79] Furthermore, although parietal hypometabolism/perfusion can be a feature in DLB as it is in AD, the additional presence of occipital hypometabolism[80] or hypoperfusion[81] can aid in distinguishing DLB from AD. More recently, several radioligands for use in SPECT have been developed that bind to the dopamine reuptake or transporter site. Low radiotracer uptake in the caudate and putamen is a feature that distinguishes DLB from AD,[81–83] and this finding correlates with autopsy diagnosis[83]; however, reduced tracer uptake does not distinguish DLB from PD or PD with dementia,[81] and DLB and AD frequently coexist.[84]

TEMPORAL EVOLUTION OF BIOMARKERS

AD is a dynamic process and the various biomarkers do not reach abnormal levels or maxima at the same time; they vary with the stages of the pathophysiologic process.[85] From a hypothetical sequence of events proposed by Jack and colleagues,[85] as shown in **Fig. 5**, the initiating process in the AD cascade involves the deposition of amyloid in the brain, typically during the preclinical stage. The precise timing of this relative to the subsequent presentation of clinical symptoms is not known, but the construct of the initiating event being amyloid deposition is well documented.[86] Thus, in vivo markers of amyloid deposition, including amyloid PET imaging and CSF $A\beta_{42}$, are likely to be

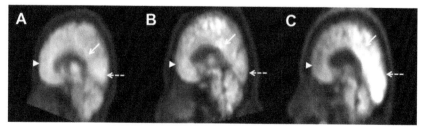

Fig. 4. Comparison of FDG-PET in AD, DLB, and frontotemporal dementia (FTD). Sagittal section of FDG-PET scans in individuals with AD (*A*), DLB (*B*), and FTD (*C*). AD is characterized by temporoparietal and posterior cingulate hypometabolism (*A, white arrow*) relative to other cortical areas, whereas occipital hypometabolism is noted in DLB (*B, dashed arrow*), and frontal hypometabolism is apparent in FTD (*C, arrowhead*).

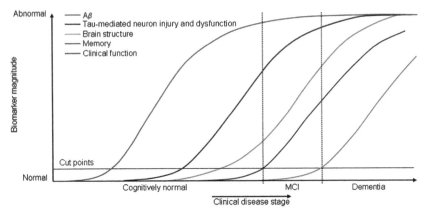

Fig. 5. The theoretic evolution of biomarkers in the Alzheimer pathologic cascade. Amyloid deposition is the initiating event in the pathologic cascade and corresponding biomarkers (low CSF Aβ declines and positive amyloid imaging) are detected before the development of clinical symptoms. As neurodegeneration occurs, evidence of brain dysfunction can be measured through CSF tau levels, FDG-PET, or SPECT. As memory and clinical function decline, structural brain MRI changes are noted. (*Modified from* Jack CR Jr, Knopman DS, Jagust WJ, et al. Hypothetical model of dynamic biomarkers of the Alzheimer's pathological cascade. Lancet Neurol 2010;9:119–28.)

abnormal before the presence of clinical symptoms. Between 20% and 40% of cognitively normal elderly have abnormal amyloid imaging or CSF Aβ$_{42}$ levels, with a similar proportion having a pathologic diagnosis of AD despite no clinical symptoms.[85] Serial PiB imaging scans have suggested that amyloid may begin accumulating as many as 15 to 20 years before the presence of clinical symptoms.[87,88] By the time clinical symptoms appear, PiB retention rates and CSF Aβ$_{42}$ levels have largely saturated and do not correlate with cognitive decline.[22,23,87,89,90]

Following the deposition of amyloid, there is a sequence of events characterizing neurodegeneration that leads to the appearance of abnormal biomarkers of neurodegeneration, including MRI, FDG-PET, SPECT, and CSF tau.[85] However, the appearance of abnormalities of these markers is likely also temporally ordered. FDG-PET hypometabolism and increased CSF tau may precede MRI changes because it is these MRI changes that correlate best with clinical impairment in MCI and AD.[91,92] As depicted in **Fig. 5**, it is only after these events take place that clinical symptoms evolve. Memory impairment is typically the first symptom to develop, characterizing the typical MCI stage. As the disease progresses, other cognitive domains become impaired and daily function is compromised, leading to dementia.

As is also depicted in **Fig. 5**, none of the biomarkers are static, but the rate of change of each biomarker varies over the course of disease progression.[85,93] The dynamic changes are easiest to appreciate in imaging modalities, providing an advantage for these biomarkers compared with CSF (see **Figs. 2** and **3**). For example, cerebral atrophy begins in the medial temporal lobes and spreads outward to the limbic and paralimbic areas and later the isocortical association areas.[94] Thus, as depicted in **Fig. 5** from the hypothetical model of AD by Jack and colleagues,[85] FDG-PET abnormalities in the precuneus and posterior cingulate precede changes in the lateral temporal and frontal areas, with a similar pattern occurring with changes in structural MRI.[85]

Given the dynamic nature of the biomarkers, the presence, absence, or intensity of biomarkers can aid in disease staging and prognostication. For example, a cognitively normal elderly individual is expected to have abnormal amyloid imaging and low CSF $A\beta_{42}$ if that individual is going to develop AD. An individual with early MCI caused by AD likewise has abnormal amyloid imaging and low CSF $A\beta_{42}$, whereas CSF tau may be modestly increased and brain structure on MRI appears normal. As clinical symptoms become more apparent in later stages of MCI and early dementia, levels of CSF tau become definitively increased and rates of brain atrophy begin to increase rapidly.

This model has proved to be useful in aging and dementia for characterizing putative pathologic processes and their sequences. However, the precise temporal ordering of these events, the shapes of the curves, and the thresholds for what is normal and abnormal on each of these markers are largely unknown.

APPLICATION

The combination of a clinical syndrome and biomarker information can result in varying levels of certainty about the underlying process. In a patient with MCI, evidence of both $A\beta$ deposition and neuronal injury confers the highest likelihood that the pathophysiologic process is caused by AD. Under that hypothesis, new research criteria for the diagnosis of MCI, using biomarker data, have been proposed[9]:

MCI: Core Clinical Criteria

An individual meets core clinical criteria for MCI but:

1. No biomarker information is available
2. Biomarkers conflict with one another
3. Biomarker results are indeterminate (neither clearly positive nor negative)

MCI Caused by AD: Intermediate Likelihood

An individual meets core clinical criteria for MCI with either:

1. Positive biomarkers reflecting $A\beta$ deposition but biomarkers of neuronal injury have not or cannot be tested.
   or
2. Positive biomarkers reflecting neuronal injury but biomarkers of $A\beta$ deposition have not or cannot be tested.

MCI Caused by AD: High Likelihood

An individual meets core clinical criteria for MCI and also has positive biomarkers reflecting $A\beta$ deposition (positive PET amyloid imaging or low CSF $A\beta_{42}$) and neuronal injury (structural MRI changes, increased CSF tau, or hypometabolism/perfusion in the posterior temporoparietal regions).

MCI: Unlikely to be Caused by AD

An individual meets core clinical criteria for MCI but has negative biomarkers reflecting $A\beta$ deposition and neuronal injury. An alternate cause of MCI should be sought.

LIMITATIONS

The research evaluating the use of biomarkers and their clinical applications are has pitfalls (**Box 1**). Many studies are in select research populations and not routine clinical populations.[27] Likewise, most study participants are clinically diagnosed, which means that the performance of the biomarkers in those studies cannot be higher than the clinical criteria used.[27] For example, clinical criteria often do not account for coexisting AD disorders in cognitively impaired subjects[95,96] or control subjects

> **Box 1**
> **Limitations of biomarkers for AD**
>
> 1. Most studies performed in select research populations
> 2. Lack of validation in autopsy studies
> 3. Lack of data for follow-up past 1 to 2 years
> 4. Difficulty in collecting, processing, and interpreting CSF biomarker data
> 5. Nonspecificity of biomarkers
> 6. Precise temporal evolution of biomarkers not known

with asymptomatic AD disorders[97]; it is therefore unclear whether suboptimal diagnostic performance of biomarkers is related to the biomarkers or the populations in which they were studied.[27]

Furthermore, many studies assessing the usefulness of biomarkers as indicators of progression from MCI to dementia have been completed over a follow-up period of 1 to 2 years. However, the conversion rate of MCI to dementia is approximately 10% to 15% per year.[98–100] A longer follow-up period is therefore needed to determine the usefulness of biomarkers in slow or nonprogressive individuals.[27]

There is also a great deal of difficulty for the practicing physician in collecting, processing, and interpreting CSF biomarkers. A lumbar puncture is invasive, and may be avoided because of fear of patient discomfort or complications. When collecting CSF, nonabsorbent polypropylene test tubes are needed to prevent the $A\beta_{42}$ or tau proteins from binding to the tube walls and falsely lowering the results.[27] In addition, although there is an international standardization exercise underway sponsored by the Alzheimer's Association to bring multiple laboratories together to standardize CSF collection and assay methodology, there is currently not a standard cutoff threshold for CSF measures.

In addition, despite significant gains in research, a great deal of uncertainty remains in the test results of the biomarkers. First, the biomarkers are not specific for AD. Positive amyloid imaging can be seen in cerebral amyloid angiopathy[101,102]; low CSF $A\beta_{42}$ can be seen in DLB,[103] frontotemporal dementia, vascular dementia,[66] Creutzfeldt-Jakob disease,[104] amyotrophic lateral sclerosis,[105] or multiple system atrophy[106]; increased CSF tau can be found in stroke, traumatic brain injury, or prion diseases.[67–69] Second, despite the great usefulness of Jack and colleagues[85] model of biomarkers in the AD cascade, the precise temporal ordering of events, shapes of the curves, and thresholds for normal and abnormal is unknown.[85] For instance, the lag phase between amyloid deposition and appearance of neuronal degeneration remains to be elucidated. It is also common for biomarker results to conflict, and the exact interpretation of the data in this circumstance is unknown.

EMERGING BIOMARKERS

Several other measures, including other CSF and imaging studies, as well as blood assays, are being considered as potential biomarkers but have yet to be approved for clinical practice (**Table 3**). For example, CSF levels of visininlike protein-1 (VILIP-1), a neuronal calcium-sensor protein, has shown usefulness as a marker of neuronal injury in brain injury models,[107] and CSF VILIP-1 and VILIP-1/Aβ42 predict rates of global cognitive decline similarly to tau and tau/Aβ42 in individuals with very mild or mild AD.[108]

Table 3 Emerging biomarkers	
Purpose	Biomarker
Marker of amyloid disorders in AD	Plasma $A\beta_{42}$
Marker of synapse dysfunction and neurodegeneration in AD	CSF VILIP-1 Hydrogen 1 MR spectroscopy Functional MRI Diffusion tensor imaging MR perfusion
Marker of oxidative stress and inflammation	CSF isoprostane CSF interleukins and growth factors CSF S-100B and GFAP CSF YKL-40
Lipidomics	Serum ceramides
Marker of non-AD process	CSF alpha-synuclein CSF neurofilament CSF TDP-43

Abbreviations: GFAP, glial fibrillary acidic protein; TDP-43, TAR DNA-binding protein 43; VILIP, visininlike protein; YSL-40, Chitinase-3-like protein 1.

Plasma Aβ

Given the invasive nature of obtaining CSF, a blood marker for amyloid deposition is ideal to identify and treat presymptomatic or early symptomatic individuals. Several studies have investigated plasma measures of $A\beta_{42}$ and $A\beta_{40}$ for early biomarkers of AD disorders. However, results thus far have been inconsistent with a recent systematic review and meta-analysis not showing a significant correlation with plasma levels of $A\beta_{42}$ and $A\beta_{40}$ alone and risk of AD or dementia, although $A\beta_{42}/A\beta_{40}$ ratios were suggestive.[12] Lack of standardized assays and longitudinal studies across all stages of cognitive function have also limited the usefulness of this biomarker.

Markers of Oxidative Stress and Inflammation

AD is associated with an inflammatory reaction and oxidative stress. Several studies have assessed CSF measures of these processes. Isoprostane, a marker of oxidative stress, is the most widely studied and increases early in the course of AD disorders and may increase diagnostic accuracy in MCI.[109,110] S-100B and Glial Fibrillary Acidic Protein (GFAP), as markers of astrocytic activity and gliosis, and several interleukins and growth factors, as markers of the inflammatory response, have been studied, but data on their usefulness has been inconclusive.[111] Chitinase-3-like protein 1 (YKL-40), a glycoprotein with sequence homology to bacterial and fungal chitinases and chitin binding ability, is involved in inflammation and tissue remodeling and is increased in AD; a combination of CSF levels of YKL-40 and $A\beta_{42}$ predicts risk of developing cognitive impairment in preclinical AD.[112] Likewise, there continues to be interest in developing peripheral blood markers for these processes, but this has been hampered by the short half-life, lack of correlation between CSF and peripheral blood levels, and association of many of these markers with normal aging.[113]

Lipidomics

Lipids seem to play a crucial role in AD disorders because the brain is composed of 20% lipids, more than any other organ, and the ε4 allele of apolipoprotein E (ApoE), which plays a role in lipid processing and transport, increased susceptibility to late onset AD. Two classes of lipids, glycerophospholipids and sphingolipids, have been most studied.[114] Certain serum ceramides (metabolites of sphingomyelin) may predict development of AD and, less so, all-cause dementia in cognitively normal women,[115] and may also predict cognitive loss and right hippocampal volume loss in MCI.[116]

Hydrogen 1 MR Spectroscopy

Dementing illnesses can affect levels of different brain metabolites, including N-acetylaspartate (NAA), choline (cho), myoinositol (mi), and creatine (Cr). For example, N-acetylaspartate (NAA) is a measure of neuronal integrity and is reduced in the cortical gray and white matter in patients with AD, corresponding with areas of significant neurofibrillary tangle deposition. The NAA/Cr ratio is therefore decreased in the posterior cingulate gyrus, an area involved early in AD disorders, but is normal in the occipital lobe, an area without significant tangles until later in the disease course.[117] In contrast, choline and myoinositol peaks are increased in AD, perhaps related to increased phosphatidylcholine catabolism or downregulation of choline acetyltransferase and activated glial cells around amyloid plaques in AD, respectively.[118] In single-domain amnestic MCI, mi/Cr ratios are increased similarly to AD, whereas mi/Cr ratios are more likely to be normal in nonamnestic MCI, suggesting the contribution of cerebrovascular disease or other neurodegenerative diseases to the cognitive impairment.[119]

Disease-specific spectroscopic patterns have been noted and thus MR spectroscopy (MRS) can aid in diagnosis. Although frontotemporal dementia has a similar pattern to AD (decreased NAA/Cr ratio and increased mi/Cr ratio),[120] vascular dementia is associated with a low NAA/Cr ratio in the posterior cingulate, but normal mi/Cr ratio. Increased mi/Cr ratio in a demented individual with significant vascular burden may therefore suggest coexisting AD disorders.[121,122] In contrast, DLB is associated with normal NAA/Cr ratio in the posterior cingulate, but increased Cho/Cr ratio.[120] However, acquisition and interpretation of MRS data is technically challenging and MRS has not yet been validated in autopsy series to permit its use in the clinical setting.

Functional MRI

Functional MRI (fMRI) modalities highlight the functional connectivity of brain networks, either at rest or task based. At rest, blood oxygen level–dependent (BOLD) signal intrinsically fluctuates; brain networks that are functionally connected theoretically show synchronous temporal fluctuations.[123] The brain networks that are active at rest, the default mode network, include the hippocampus, posterior cingulate, precuneus, parietal cortex, and medial prefrontal cortex. Because these areas are involved early in AD disorders, resting fMRI in AD and MCI shows corresponding decrease in the default mode.[124] In task-based fMRI, demented individuals show decreased activation, whereas individuals with preclinical disorders and MCI show increased activation, perhaps representing a compensatory state to mask functional impairment, or, alternatively, a pathologic increase contributing to cognitive decline.[124]

Diffusion Tensor Imaging

Diffusion tensor imaging (DTI) is a measure of structural connectivity under the principle that water molecules diffuse preferentially along the axon. As AD disorders disrupt cell membranes and thus diffusion of water molecules, the mean diffusivity (MD) is increased and the directional water diffusivity, or fractional anisotropy, is decreased along white matter tracts connecting affected areas of brain, including the medial temporal lobes and posterior cingulate.[124] Fractional anisotropy measures can also predict conversion of MCI to dementia.[124]

MR Perfusion

Using the same hypothesis as for SPECT, MR perfusion imaging is designed to measure disease-specific regional blood flow decreases via arterial spin labeling techniques.[125,126] This modality is attractive because it allows the clinician to obtain similar information as with SPECT or FDG-PET noninvasively in the same examination with other MR modalities, but sensitivity and specificity measures are yet to be elucidated.[124,127,128]

CSF Markers of Non-AD Dementias

Alpha synuclein is the major component of Lewy bodies, the pathologic hallmark of PD and DLB. Alpha synuclein seems to be reduced in the CSF of patients with PD and DLB,[129] but alpha synuclein measurements have not reliably distinguished DLB from AD.[130–132] Likewise, CSF neurofilament levels seem to be increased in FTLD compared with early AD, but these measurements have not reliably distinguished between different dementia syndromes.[133] CSF measurements of TAR DNA-binding protein 43 (TDP-43) have also been of interest given that TDP-43 inclusions are a common abnormality in FTLD; although CSF TDP-43 levels are increased in FTLD, there is significant overlap with controls.[134]

SUMMARY

Knowledge of aging and dementia is rapidly evolving with the aim of identifying individuals in the earliest stages of disease processes. Biomarkers allow the clinician to show the presence of an underlying pathologic process and resultant synapse dysfunction and neurodegeneration, even in those earliest stages. PET amyloid imaging and CSF $A\beta_{42}$ provide direct evidence of amyloid deposition and structural MRI, FDG-PET or SPECT, and CSF tau provide indirect evidence of synapse dysfunction and neurodegeneration when the pathologic process is caused by AD. Structural MRI, FDG-PET or SPECT, and PET with dopamine ligands are also valuable in establishing non-AD pathologic processes. Although these biomarkers are useful and can even be applied to diagnostic criteria in MCI, several limitations exist. Several new biomarkers are emerging and a more biological characterization of underlying pathophysiologic spectra may become possible, which could translate into earlier and more definitive clinical diagnosis and treatment.

REFERENCES

1. Jack CR Jr, Knopman DS, Weigand SD, et al. An operational approach to NIA-AA criteria for preclinical Alzheimer's disease. Ann Neurol 2012;71(6):765–75.
2. Knopman DS, Jack CR Jr, Wiste HJ, et al. Short-term clinical outcomes for stages of NIA-AA preclinical Alzheimer disease. Neurology 2012;78:1576–82.
3. Sperling RA, Aisen PS, Beckett LA, et al. Toward defining the preclinical stages of Alzheimer's disease: recommendations from the National Institute on Aging-Alzheimer's Association workgroups on diagnostic guidelines for Alzheimer's disease. Alzheimers Dement 2011;7:280–92.
4. Petersen RC, Smith GE, Waring SC, et al. Mild cognitive impairment: clinical characterization and outcome. Arch Neurol 1999;56:303–8.
5. Petersen RC. Mild cognitive impairment as a diagnostic entity. J Intern Med 2004;256:183–94.

6. DeCarli C. Mild cognitive impairment: prevalence, prognosis, aetiology, and treatment. Lancet Neurol 2003;2:15–21.

7. Gauthier S, Reisberg B, Zaudig M, et al. Mild cognitive impairment. Lancet 2006;367:1262–70.

8. Winblad B, Palmer K, Kivipelto M, et al. Mild cognitive impairment - beyond controversies, towards a consensus. J Intern Med 2004;256:240–6.

9. Albert MS, DeKosky ST, Dickson D, et al. The diagnosis of mild cognitive impairment due to Alzheimer's disease: recommendations from the National Institute on Aging and Alzheimer's Association Workgroup. Alzheimers Dement 2011;7:270–9.

10. Hyman BT, Phelps CH, Beach TG, et al. National Institute on Aging-Alzheimer's Association guidelines for the neuropathologic assessment of Alzheimer's disease. Alzheimers Dement 2012;8:1–13.

11. Clark CM, Schneider JA, Bedell BJ, et al. Use of florbetapir-PET for imaging B-amyloid pathology. JAMA 2011;305:275–83.

12. Koyama A, Okereke OI, Yang T, et al. Plasma amyloid-beta as a predictor of dementia and cognitive decline: a systematic review and meta-analysis. Arch Neurol 2012;69(7):824–31.

13. Klunk WE, Engler H, Nordberg A, et al. Imaging brain amyloid in Alzheimer's disease with Pittsburgh compound-B. Ann Neurol 2004;55:306–19.

14. Wong DF, Rosenberg PB, Zhou Y, et al. In vivo imaging of amyloid deposition in Alzheimer disease using the radioligand 18F-AV-45 (florbetapir [corrected] F 18). J Nucl Med 2010;51:913–20.

15. Kemppainen NM, Aalto S, Wilson IA, et al. Voxel-based analysis of PET amyloid ligand [11C]PIB uptake in Alzheimer disease. Neurology 2006;67:1575–80.

16. Chetelat G, Villemagne VL, Pike KE, et al. Independent contribution of temporal beta-amyloid deposition to memory decline in the pre-dementia phase of Alzheimer's disease. Brain 2011;134:798–807.

17. Bacskai BJ, Frosch MP, Freeman SH, et al. Molecular imaging with Pittsburgh compound B confirmed at autopsy: a case report. Arch Neurol 2007;64:431–4.

18. Ikonomovic MD, Klunk WE, Abrahamson EE, et al. Post-mortem correlates of in vivo PiB-PET amyloid imaging in a typical case of Alzheimer's disease. Brain 2008;131:1630–45.

19. Rosen RF, Ciliax BJ, Wingo TS, et al. Deficient high-affinity binding of Pittsburgh compound B in a case of Alzheimer's disease. Acta Neuropathol 2010;119(2):221–33.

20. Wolk DA, Price JC, Saxton JA, et al. Amyloid imaging in mild cognitive impairment subtypes. Ann Neurol 2009;65:557–68.

21. Villemagne VL, Pike KE, Chetelat G, et al. Longitudinal assessment of Abeta and cognition in aging and Alzheimer disease. Ann Neurol 2011;69:181–92.

22. Doraiswamy PM, Sperling RA, Coleman RE, et al. Amyloid-beta assessed by florbetapir F 18 PET and 18-month cognitive decline: a multicenter study. Neurology 2012;79:1636–44.

23. Landau SM, Mintun MA, Joshi AD, et al. Amyloid deposition, hypometabolism, and longitudinal cognitive decline. Ann Neurol 2012;72(4):578–86.

24. Jack CR Jr, Wiste HJ, Vemuri P, et al. Brain beta-amyloid measures and magnetic resonance imaging atrophy both predict time-to-progression from mild cognitive impairment to Alzheimer's disease. Brain 2010;133:3336–48.

25. Strozyk D, Blennow K, White LR, et al. CSF Abeta 42 levels correlate with amyloid-neuropathology in a population-based autopsy study. Neurology 2003;60:652–6.

26. Clark CM, Xie S, Chittams J, et al. Cerebrospinal fluid tau and beta-amyloid: how well do these biomarkers reflect autopsy-confirmed dementia diagnoses? Arch Neurol 2003;60:1696–702.
27. Blennow K, Hampel H. CSF markers for incipient Alzheimer's disease. Lancet Neurol 2003;2:605–13.
28. Hansson O, Zetterberg H, Buchhave P, et al. Association between CSF biomarkers and incipient Alzheimer's disease in patients with mild cognitive impairment: a follow-up study. Lancet Neurol 2006;5:228–34.
29. Mattsson N, Zetterberg H, Hansson O, et al. CSF biomarkers and incipient Alzheimer disease in patients with mild cognitive impairment. JAMA 2009;302:385–93.
30. Riemenschneider M, Lautenschlager N, Wagenpfeil S, et al. Cerebrospinal fluid tau and beta-amyloid 42 proteins identify Alzheimer disease in subjects with mild cognitive impairment. Arch Neurol 2002;59:1729–34.
31. Fagan AM, Mintun MA, Mach RH, et al. Inverse relation between in vivo amyloid imaging load and cerebrospinal fluid Abeta42 in humans. Ann Neurol 2006;59:512–9.
32. Jagust WJ, Landau SM, Shaw LM, et al. Relationships between biomarkers in aging and dementia. Neurology 2009;73:1193–9.
33. Grimmer T, Riemenschneider M, Forstl H, et al. Beta amyloid in Alzheimer's disease: increased deposition in brain is reflected in reduced concentration in cerebrospinal fluid. Biol Psychiatry 2009;65:927–34.
34. Tolboom N, van der Flier WM, Yaqub M, et al. Relationship of cerebrospinal fluid markers to 11C-PiB and 18F-FDDNP binding. J Nucl Med 2009;50:1464–70.
35. Terry RD, Masliah E, Salmon DP, et al. Physical basis of cognitive alterations in Alzheimer's disease: synapse loss is the major correlate of cognitive impairment. Ann Neurol 1991;30:572–80.
36. Apostolova LG, Dutton RA, Dinov ID, et al. Conversion of mild cognitive impairment to Alzheimer disease predicted by hippocampal atrophy maps. Arch Neurol 2006;63:693–9.
37. Jack CR, Weigand SD, Shiung MM, et al. Atrophy rates accelerate in amnestic mild cognitive impairment. Neurology 2008;70:1740–52.
38. Bobinski M, de Leon MJ, Wegiel J, et al. The histological validation of post mortem magnetic resonance imaging-determined hippocampal volume in Alzheimer's disease. Neuroscience 2000;95:721–5.
39. Jack CR, Petersen RC, Xu YC, et al. Prediction of AD with MRI-based hippocampal volume in mild cognitive impairment. Neurology 1999;52:1397–403.
40. Bakkour A, Morris JC, Dickerson BC. The cortical signature of prodromal AD: regional thinning predicts mild AD dementia. Neurology 2009;72:1048–55.
41. van de Pol LA, van der Flier WM, Korf ES, et al. Baseline predictors of rates of hippocampal atrophy in mild cognitive impairment. Neurology 2007;69:1491–7.
42. Fischl B, Salat DH, Busa E, et al. Whole brain segmentation: automated labeling of neuroanatomical structures in the human brain. Neuron 2002;33:341–55.
43. Jack C, Barkhof F, Bernstein M, et al. Steps to standardization and validation of hippocampal volumetry as a biomarker in clinical trials and diagnostic criteria for Alzheimer's disease. Alzheimers Dement 2011;7(4):474–85.
44. Attwell D, Laughlin SB. An energy budget for signaling in the grey matter of the brain. J Cereb Blood Flow Metab 2001;21:1133–45.
45. Schwartz WJ, Smith CB, Davidsen L, et al. Metabolic mapping of functional activity in the hypothalamo-neurohypophysial system of the rat. Science 1979;205:723–5.

46. Jagust W, Reed B, Mungas D, et al. What does fluorodeoxyglucose PET imaging add to a clinical diagnosis of dementia? Neurology 2007;69:871–7.

47. Hoffman JM, Welsh-Bohmer KA, Hanson M, et al. FDG PET imaging in patients with pathologically verified dementia. J Nucl Med 2000;41:1920–8.

48. Ibanez V, Pietrini P, Alexander GE, et al. Regional glucose metabolic abnormalities are not the result of atrophy in Alzheimer's disease. Neurology 1998;50: 1585–93.

49. Reiman EM, Caselli RJ, Lang S, et al. Preclinical evidence of Alzheimer's disease in persons homozygous for the E4 allele for apolipoprotein E. N Engl J Med 1996;334:752–8.

50. Reiman EM, Caselli RJ, Chen K, et al. Declining brain activity in cognitively normal apolipoprotein E epsilon 4 heterozygotes: a foundation for using positron emission tomography to efficiently test treatments to prevent Alzheimer's disease. Proc Natl Acad Sci U S A 2001;98:3334–9.

51. Chetelat G, Desgranges B, de la Sayette V, et al. Mild cognitive impairment: can FDG-PET predict who is to rapidly convert to Alzheimer's disease? Neurology 2003;60:1374–7.

52. Landau SM, Harvey D, Madison CM, et al. Comparing predictors of conversion and decline in mild cognitive impairment. Neurology 2010;75:230–8.

53. Jagust W, Budinger TF, Reed BR. The diagnosis of dementia with single photon emission computed tomography. Arch Neurol 1987;44:258–62.

54. Kanetaka H, Matsuda H, Asada T, et al. Effects of partial volume correction on discrimination between very early Alzheimer's dementia and controls using brain perfusion SPECT. Eur J Nucl Med Mol Imaging 2004;31:975–80.

55. Bradley KM, O'Sullivan VT, Soper ND, et al. Cerebral perfusion SPET correlated with Braak pathological stage in Alzheimer's disease. Brain 2002;125:1772–81.

56. Borroni B, Anchisi D, Paghera B, et al. Combined 99mTc-ECD SPECT and neuropsychological studies in MCI for the assessment of conversion to AD. Neurobiol Aging 2006;27:24–31.

57. Hirao K, Ohnishi T, Hirata Y, et al. The prediction of rapid conversion to Alzheimer's disease in mild cognitive impairment using regional cerebral blood flow SPECT. Neuroimage 2005;28:1014–21.

58. Herholz K, Schopphoff H, Schmidt M, et al. Direct comparison of spatially normalized PET and SPECT scans in Alzheimer's disease. J Nucl Med 2002; 43:21–6.

59. Messa C, Perani D, Lucignani G, et al. High-resolution technetium-99m-HMPAO SPECT in patients with probable Alzheimer's disease: comparison with fluorine-18-FDG PET. J Nucl Med 1994;35:210–6.

60. Arai H, Terajima M, Miura M, et al. Tau in cerebrospinal fluid: a potential diagnostic marker in Alzheimer's disease. Ann Neurol 1995;38:649–52.

61. Blennow K, Wallin A, Agren H, et al. Tau protein in cerebrospinal fluid: a biochemical marker for axonal degeneration in Alzheimer disease? Mol Chem Neuropathol 1995;26:231–45.

62. Tapiola T, Overmyer M, Lehtovirta M, et al. The level of cerebrospinal fluid tau correlates with neurofibrillary tangles in Alzheimer's disease. Neuroreport 1997;8:3961–3.

63. Jagust W, Thisted R, Devous MD, et al. SPECT perfusion imaging in the diagnosis of Alzheimer's disease: a clinical-pathologic study. Neurology 2001;56: 950–6.

64. Andreasen N, Minthon L, Clarberg A, et al. Sensitivity, specificity, and stability of CSF-tau in AD in a community-based patient sample. Neurology 1999;53:1488–94.

65. Morikawa YI, Arai H, Matsushita S, et al. Cerebrospinal fluid tau protein levels in demented and nondemented alcoholics. Alcohol Clin Exp Res 1999;23: 575–7.

66. Sjögren M, Minthon L, Davidsson P, et al. CSF levels of tau, β-amyloid 1-42 and GAP-43 in frontotemporal dementia, other types of dementia and normal aging. J Neural Transm 2000;107:563–79.

67. Hesse C, Rosengren L, Andreasen N, et al. Transient increase in total tau but not phospho-tau in human cerebrospinal fluid after acute stroke. Neurosci Lett 2001;297:187–90.

68. Ost M, Nylen K, Csajbok L, et al. Initial CSF total tau correlates with 1-year outcome in patients with traumatic brain injury. Neurology 2006;67:1600–4.

69. Otto M, Wiltfang J, Cepek L, et al. Tau protein and 14-3-3 protein in the differential diagnosis of Creutzfeldt-Jakob disease. Neurology 2002;58:192–7.

70. Grundke-Iqbal I, Iqbal K, Tung YC, et al. Abnormal phosphorylation of the microtubule-associated protein tau (tau) in Alzheimer cytoskeletal pathology. Proc Natl Acad Sci U S A 1986;83:4913–7.

71. Riemenschneider M, Wagenpfeil S, Vanderstichele H, et al. Phospho-tau//total tau ratio in cerebrospinal fluid discriminates Creutzfeldt-Jakob disease from other dementias. Mol Psychiatry 2003;8:343–7.

72. Sjogren M, Davidsson P, Tullberg M, et al. Both total and phosphorylated tau are increased in Alzheimer's disease. J Neurol Neurosurg Psychiatry 2001;70: 624–30.

73. Parnetti L, Lanari A, Amici S, et al. CSF phosphorylated tau is a possible marker for discriminating Alzheimer's disease from dementia with Lewy bodies. Neurol Sci 2001;22:77–8.

74. Herukka SK, Hallikainen M, Soininen H, et al. CSF Abeta42 and tau or phosphorylated tau and prediction of progressive mild cognitive impairment. Neurology 2005;64:1294–7.

75. Van Rossum IA, Vos S, Handels R, et al. Biomarkers as predictors for conversion from mild cognitive impairment to Alzheimer-type dementia: implications for trial design. J Alzheimers Dis 2010;20:881–91.

76. Jeong Y, Cho SS, Park JM, et al. 18F-FDG PET Findings in frontotemporal dementia: an SPM analysis of 29 patients. J Nucl Med 2005;46:233–9.

77. Foster NL, Heidebrink JL, Clark CM, et al. FDG-PET improves accuracy in distinguishing frontotemporal dementia and Alzheimer's disease. Brain 2007;130: 2616–35.

78. McNeill R, Sare GM, Manoharan M, et al. Accuracy of single-photon emission computed tomography in differentiating frontotemporal dementia from Alzheimer's disease. J Neurol Neurosurg Psychiatry 2007;78:350–5.

79. Taylor KI, Probst A, Miserez AR, et al. Clinical course of neuropathologically confirmed frontal-variant Alzheimer's disease. Nat Clin Pract Neurol 2008;4: 226–32.

80. Minoshima S, Foster NL, Sima AA, et al. Alzheimer's disease versus dementia with Lewy bodies: cerebral metabolic distinction with autopsy confirmation. Ann Neurol 2001;50:358–65.

81. O'Brien J, Colloby S, Fenwick J, et al. Dopamine transporter loss visualized with FP-CIT SPECT in the differential diagnosis of dementia with Lewy bodies. Arch Neurol 2004;61:919–25.

82. McKeith I, O'Brien J, Walker Z, et al. Sensitivity and specificity of dopamine transporter imaging with 123I-FP-CIT SPECT in dementia with Lewy bodies: a phase III, multicentre study. Lancet Neurol 2007;6:305–13.

83. Walker Z, Costa DC, Walker RW, et al. Differentiation of dementia with Lewy bodies from Alzheimer's disease using a dopaminergic presynaptic ligand. J Neurol Neurosurg Psychiatry 2002;73:134–40.

84. Hansen LA, Samuel W. Criteria for Alzheimer's disease and the nosology of dementia with Lewy bodies. Neurology 1997;48:126–32.

85. Jack C Jr, Knopman D, Jagust W, et al. Hypothetical model of dynamic biomarkers of the Alzheimer's pathological cascade. Lancet Neurol 2010;9:119–28.

86. Hardy J, Selkoe DJ. The amyloid hypothesis of Alzheimer's disease: progress and problems on the road to therapeutics. Science 2002;297:353–6.

87. Jack C Jr, Low V, Weigand S, et al. Serial PiB and MRI in normal, mild cognitive impairment and Alzheimer's disease: implications for sequence of pathological events in Alzheimer's disease. Brain 2009;132:1355–65.

88. Jack CR, Wiste HJ, Lesnick TG, et al. Brain β-amyloid load approaches a plateau. Neurology 2013;80(10):890–6.

89. Buchhave P, Minthon L, Zetterberg H, et al. Cerebrospinal fluid levels of beta-amyloid 1-42, but not of tau, are fully changed already 5 to 10 years before the onset of Alzheimer dementia. Arch Gen Psychiatry 2012;69:98–106.

90. Engler H, Forsberg A, Almkvist O, et al. Two-year follow-up of amyloid deposition in patients with Alzheimer's disease. Brain 2006;129:2856–66.

91. Vemuri P, Wiste HJ, Weigand SD, et al. MRI and CSF biomarkers in normal, MCI, and AD subjects: predicting future clinical change. Neurology 2009;73:294–301.

92. Fox NC, Freeborough PA. Brain atrophy progression measured from registered serial MRI: validation and application to Alzheimer's disease. J Magn Reson Imaging 1997;7:1069–75.

93. Wahlund LO, Blennow K. Cerebrospinal fluid biomarkers for disease stage and intensity in cognitively impaired patients. Neurosci Lett 2003;339:99–102.

94. Whitwell JL, Przybelski SA, Weigand SD, et al. 3D maps from multiple MRI illustrate changing atrophy patterns as subjects progress from mild cognitive impairment to Alzheimer's disease. Brain 2007;130:1777–86.

95. Galasko D, Hansen LA, Katzman R, et al. Clinical-neuropathological correlations in Alzheimer's disease and related dementias. Arch Neurol 1994;51:888–95.

96. Jellinger KA. Diagnostic accuracy of Alzheimer's disease: a clinicopathological study. Acta Neuropathol 1996;91:219–20.

97. Price JL, Morris JC. Tangles and plaques in nondemented aging and "preclinical" Alzheimer's disease. Ann Neurol 1999;45:358–68.

98. Lopez OL, Jagust WJ, DeKosky ST, et al. Prevalence and classification of mild cognitive impairment in the cardiovascular health study cognition study. Arch Neurol 2003;60:1385–9.

99. Ganguli M, Dodge HH, Shen C, et al. Mild cognitive impairment, amnestic type: an epidemiologic study. Neurology 2004;63:115–21.

100. Petersen RC, Roberts RO, Knopman DS, et al. Prevalence of mild cognitive impairment is higher in men: the Mayo Clinic study of aging. Neurology 2010;75:889–97.

101. Ly JV, Donnan GA, Villemagne VL, et al. 11C-PIB binding is increased in patients with cerebral amyloid angiopathy-related hemorrhage. Neurology 2010;74:487–93.

102. Johnson KA, Gregas M, Becker JA, et al. Imaging of amyloid burden and distribution in cerebral amyloid angiopathy. Ann Neurol 2007;62:229–34.

103. Kanemaru K, Kameda N, Yamanouchi H. Decreased CSF amyloid beta42 and normal tau levels in dementia with Lewy bodies. Neurology 2000;54:1875–6.

104. Otto M, Esselmann H, Schulz-Shaeffer W, et al. Decreased beta-amyloid1-42 in cerebrospinal fluid of patients with Creutzfeldt-Jakob disease. Neurology 2000; 54:1099–102.

105. Sjogren M, Davidsson P, Wallin A, et al. Decreased CSF-beta-amyloid 42 in Alzheimer's disease and amyotrophic lateral sclerosis may reflect mismetabolism of beta-amyloid induced by disparate mechanisms. Dement Geriatr Cogn Disord 2002;13:112–8.

106. Holmberg B, Johnels B, Blennow K, et al. Cerebrospinal fluid Abeta42 is reduced in multiple system atrophy but normal in Parkinson's disease and progressive supranuclear palsy. Mov Disord 2003;18:186–90.

107. Laterza OF, Modur VR, Crimmins DL, et al. Identification of novel brain biomarkers. Clin Chem 2006;52:1713–21.

108. Tarawneh R, Lee JM, Ladenson JH, et al. CSF VILIP-1 predicts rates of cognitive decline in early Alzheimer disease. Neurology 2012;78:709–19.

109. de Leon MJ, DeSanti S, Zinkowski R, et al. Longitudinal CSF and MRI biomarkers improve the diagnosis of mild cognitive impairment. Neurobiol Aging 2006;27:394–401.

110. de Leon MJ, Mosconi L, Li J, et al. Longitudinal CSF isoprostane and MRI atrophy in the progression to AD. J Neurol 2007;254:1666–75.

111. Drago V, Babiloni C, Bartres-Faz D, et al. Disease tracking markers for Alzheimer's disease at the prodromal (MCI) stage. J Alzheimers Dis 2011; 26(Suppl 3):159–99.

112. Craig-Schapiro R, Perrin RJ, Roe CM, et al. YKL-40: a novel prognostic fluid biomarker for preclinical Alzheimer's disease. Biol Psychiatry 2010;68:903–12.

113. Panza F, Solfrizzi V, Seripa D, et al. Peripheral antioxidant markers in mild cognitive impairment and its progression to dementia. J Alzheimers Dis 2010;21: 1179–83.

114. Wood PL. Lipidomics of Alzheimer's disease: current status. Alzheimers Res Ther 2012;4:5.

115. Mielke MM, Bandaru VV, Haughey NJ, et al. Serum ceramides increase the risk of Alzheimer disease: the Women's Health and Aging Study II. Neurology 2012; 79:633–41.

116. Mielke MM, Haughey NJ, Ratnam Bandaru VV, et al. Plasma ceramides are altered in mild cognitive impairment and predict cognitive decline and hippocampal volume loss. Alzheimers Dement 2010;6:378–85.

117. Kantarci K, Jack CR Jr, Xu YC, et al. Regional metabolic patterns in mild cognitive impairment and Alzheimer's disease: a 1H MRS study. Neurology 2000;55:210–7.

118. Kantarci K. 1H magnetic resonance spectroscopy in dementia. Br J Radiol 2007;80(Spec No 2):S146–52.

119. Kantarci K, Petersen RC, Przybelski SA, et al. Hippocampal volumes, proton magnetic resonance spectroscopy metabolites, and cerebrovascular disease in mild cognitive impairment subtypes. Arch Neurol 2008;65:1621–8.

120. Kantarci K, Petersen RC, Boeve BF, et al. 1H MR spectroscopy in common dementias. Neurology 2004;63:1393–8.

121. MacKay S, Meyerhoff DJ, Constans JM, et al. Regional gray and white matter metabolite differences in subjects with AD, with subcortical ischemic vascular dementia, and elderly controls with 1H magnetic resonance spectroscopic imaging. Arch Neurol 1996;53:167–74.

122. Kattapong VJ, Brooks WM, Wesley MH, et al. Proton magnetic resonance spectroscopy of vascular- and Alzheimer-type dementia. Arch Neurol 1996;53: 678–80.

123. Fox MD, Snyder AZ, Vincent JL, et al. The human brain is intrinsically organized into dynamic, anticorrelated functional networks. Proc Natl Acad Sci U S A 2005; 102:9673–8.

124. Jack CR Jr. Alzheimer disease: new concepts on its neurobiology and the clinical role imaging will play. Radiology 2012;263:344–61.

125. Alsop DC, Detre JA, Grossman M. Assessment of cerebral blood flow in Alzheimer's disease by spin-labeled magnetic resonance imaging. Ann Neurol 2000;47:93–100.

126. Du AT, Jahng GH, Hayasaka S, et al. Hypoperfusion in frontotemporal dementia and Alzheimer disease by arterial spin labeling MRI. Neurology 2006;67: 1215–20.

127. Chen Y, Wolk DA, Reddin JS, et al. Voxel-level comparison of arterial spin-labeled perfusion MRI and FDG-PET in Alzheimer disease. Neurology 2011; 77:1977–85.

128. Hu WT, Wang Z, Lee VM, et al. Distinct cerebral perfusion patterns in FTLD and AD. Neurology 2010;75:881–8.

129. Mollenhauer B, Cullen V, Kahn I, et al. Direct quantification of CSF α-synuclein by ELISA and first cross-sectional study in patients with neurodegeneration. Exp Neurol 2008;213:315–25.

130. Kasuga K, Tokutake T, Ishikawa A, et al. Differential levels of alpha-synuclein, beta-amyloid42 and tau in CSF between patients with dementia with Lewy bodies and Alzheimer's disease. J Neurol Neurosurg Psychiatry 2010;81: 608–10.

131. Noguchi-Shinohara M, Tokuda T, Yoshita M, et al. CSF alpha-synuclein levels in dementia with Lewy bodies and Alzheimer's disease. Brain Res 2009;1251:1–6.

132. Reesink FE, Lemstra AW, van Dijk KD, et al. CSF alpha-synuclein does not discriminate dementia with Lewy bodies from Alzheimer's disease. J Alzheimers Dis 2010;22:87–95.

133. de Jong D, Jansen RW, Pijnenburg YA, et al. CSF neurofilament proteins in the differential diagnosis of dementia. J Neurol Neurosurg Psychiatry 2007;78: 936–8.

134. Steinacker P, Hendrich C, Sperfeld AD, et al. TDP-43 in cerebrospinal fluid of patients with frontotemporal lobar degeneration and amyotrophic lateral sclerosis. Arch Neurol 2008;65:1481–7.

Using Neuroimaging to Inform Clinical Practice for the Diagnosis and Treatment of Mild Cognitive Impairment

Benjamin M. Hampstead, PhD[a,b],*, Gregory S. Brown, MA[a,b]

KEYWORDS

- Neuroimaging • Cognition • Mild cognitive impairment

KEY POINTS

- The general field of aging and dementia (including Geriatric Medicine, Neurology, and Neuropsychology) has benefited greatly from the synergism that exists between clinical and research settings. The literature reviewed indicates that structural neuroimaging–based measures of medial temporal lobe atrophy often correspond to objective memory impairment, may help predict conversion to dementia, and may help in developing a treatment plan for those with mild cognitive impairment (MCI).
- Although common in an elderly population, white matter hyperintensities (WMH) should not be considered benign because they have been associated with executive and memory dysfunction, and the combination of atrophy and WMH suggests more rapid progression to Alzheimer disease.
- Therefore, clinical practice could greatly benefit from the inclusion of standardized ratings of atrophy and WMH, although care is needed when selecting the exact measurement technique(s). Positron emission tomography (both metabolic and Aβ) can also meaningfully inform the diagnostic process, but clinically acquired data are likely to be of limited use when considering specific cognitive abilities.
- Functional magnetic resonance imaging has greatly informed our understanding of the widespread changes in cognitive processing that occur in those with MCI, and has also provided evidence of preserved neuroplasticity in this population.

This study was supported by the Department of Veterans Affairs, Veterans Health Administration, Office of Research and Development, and Rehabilitation Research and Development Service through grant B6366W (B.M. Hampstead). The contents of this article do not represent the views of the Department of Veterans Affairs or the United States Government. There are no conflicts of interest.
Author Contributions: Each author provided significant intellectual contribution to warrant authorship.
[a] Rehabilitation R&D Center of Excellence, Atlanta VAMC, Decatur, GA, USA; [b] Department of Rehabilitation Medicine, Emory University, Atlanta, GA, USA
* Corresponding author. Room 150, 1441 Clifton Road NE, Atlanta, GA 30322.
E-mail address: bhampst@emory.edu

Clin Geriatr Med 29 (2013) 829–845
http://dx.doi.org/10.1016/j.cger.2013.07.007
0749-0690/13/$ – see front matter Published by Elsevier Inc.

Perhaps no other area of research has benefited from the rapid development and application of structural and functional neuroimaging techniques as much as has the study of aging and dementia. In fact, the combination of these techniques has fundamentally altered our understanding of the neurobiology of Alzheimer disease (AD) because disease progression can now be examined in vivo as opposed to the sole reliance on ex vivo histopathology. Several comprehensive reviews have discussed the available imaging methods as well as benefits and challenges associated with imaging the brains of those with mild cognitive impairment (MCI) and AD, and the reader is referred to these works (eg, Rosen and colleagues[1]; see Ashford and colleagues[2] for an overview). Jack and colleagues[3] provided elegant reviews that integrate both structural and functional neuroimaging techniques as they relate to biomarkers of AD.

This review focuses on neuroimaging methods that are sensitive to change in those with MCI, especially in regard of learning and memory dysfunction, and that are likely to be available in most clinical settings. Section I discusses the most clinically relevant neuroimaging methods as they relate to cognitive functioning in MCI and AD. Key methodological issues that facilitate or impede the use of a given technique are identified. Section II provides an overview of how neuroimaging methods can improve our understanding of the neural mechanisms associated with cognitive decline. These methods can also provide evidence of preserved neuroplasticity, which is comparatively understudied in this population, yet critical for advancing treatment options.

SECTION I

The diagnosis of MCI is, by definition, a symptomatic stage that is characterized by cognitive impairment, especially in the areas of learning and memory.[4] It is therefore not surprising that neuropsychological testing accurately distinguishes healthy controls from those with even very mild AD with more than 80% sensitivity and 90% specificity, or that it accurately predicts progression to dementia.[5] These diagnostic criteria also mean clinically acquired neuroimaging is most useful for confirming (or identifying) the disease process and predicting conversion to AD. Several viable research-based techniques are included herein, each of which has the potential to provide clinically relevant information about the nature of the cognitive deficits and to help in future predictive and treatment efforts. Across all techniques, the potential for a confirmatory bias should be minimized through the use of a blinded rater.

To date, magnetic resonance imaging (MRI) and other structural neuroimaging techniques have primarily been used to rule out other potential causes for dementia (eg, stroke, neoplasm, or other structural abnormalities). However, a sufficient body of evidence now exists that structural neuroimaging can inform the clinical decision-making process in the early detection of AD and in predicting conversion from MCI to AD.

Assessment of Medial Temporal Lobe Atrophy Using Magnetic Resonance Imaging

Atrophy within the hippocampus and entorhinal cortex (EC) is frequently observed in patients with MCI, and is widely considered a biomarker for AD.[6–8] In fact, a recent meta-analysis conducted by Schroeter and colleagues[9] revealed that hippocampal and EC atrophy is characteristic of MCI, that there is greater atrophy in MCI relative to "healthy" older adults, and that atrophy in these regions is a strong predictor of conversion from MCI to AD over a 2-year period (see also Raz and Rodrigue[10]). Furthermore, atrophy in these areas is reflective of histopathologically confirmed neurofibrillary tangles of Braak stages II and III.[11] Radiologic reports often include a description of integrity of medial temporal lobe using vague terms such as "age appropriate," "mild," or "significant" to describe the degree of atrophy. These terms lack objective standards, and undoubtedly vary within and across raters and clinical context. Thus, clinical practice could be improved through the consistent and standardized use of objective measures that assess the integrity of the hippocampus and EC. However, there is no clear gold standard in this respect because several methods exist and each has its own limitations (see Chetelat and Baron[12] for a discussion of these issues). For example, visual rating scales can be relatively quick but are subjective, and interrater reliability varies depending on the scale and expertise of the rater. Volumetric analyses are time consuming but are the most accurate reflection of structural integrity; however, this accuracy depends on image resolution, specialized computer software, and analytical expertise. Brain volumes also need to be normalized (eg, using total intracranial volume) to accurately compare different individuals (see Gold and Squire[13] for a comparison of normalization methods).

Each of these approaches is reviewed briefly here (**Table 1**), but the reader should be cognizant of that no values have been identified that clearly distinguish "normal" from MCI, or MCI from AD. In fact, substantial neuronal loss is necessary before any volumetric changes occur, and it is known that cognitive reserve may allow even individuals with substantial atrophy to perform "normally."[14] Thus, quantifying atrophy can help inform the diagnosis but should be interpreted within all other clinical and neuropsychological data.

Table 1
Strengths and weaknesses of visual rating scales and volumetric measurement of the medial temporal lobes

Visual Rating Scales	Volumetric Analysis
Advantages	Advantages
Many scales are relatively quick and easy to use and show sound relationships with memory deficits	Several standardized and validated manual segmentation protocols exist for the hippocampus
Scheltens and colleagues'[15] scale has consistently demonstrated sensitivity to medial temporal atrophy in MCI and AD	Semiautomated approaches can save time and have been sensitive to structural changes in those with MCI and AD
The VRS-MTA (Duara and colleagues[20]) provides reference images to improve reliability. It consistently shows sensitivity between "healthy" elderly, MCI, and AD at the group level	Recently created, fully automated segmentation programs are capable of calculating volumetrics with relatively little user input
	Commercially available programs exist (eg, NeuroQuant) and provide basic measures that are clinically relevant. Normative data are provided. Some providers may be able to bill for the service
Disadvantages	Disadvantages
Normative data are unavailable	Normative data are typically unavailable
Reliable rating of subtle atrophy can be difficult	Manual segmentation processing time increases with resolution
Subjective nature necessitates experienced raters	Different segmentation protocols can result in up to a 2.5-fold difference in hippocampal volume
	Fully automated programs may take 24 h or more per patient (eg, FreeSurfer). More rapid, commercial programs (NeuroQuant) provide a limited number of regions

Visual rating scales

The Scheltens scale[15] is one of the most well-researched and validated visual rating scales available.[16] This scale examines hippocampal atrophy using a 5-point rating system. Atrophy ratings were originally calculated across 6 coronal sections that appeared to include a large proportion of the hippocampus (ie, slice thickness of 5 mm plus 1 mm gap, or about 30 mm total).[15] However, more recent studies have used a single, pontine-level, coronal slice that is posterior to the amygdala and mammillary bodies.[17] This evolution in the rating scale suggests that scores from earlier and more recent time periods may not be directly comparable. Regardless, this scale has repeatedly shown sensitivity to medial temporal atrophy in MCI and AD, as well as relationships between atrophy ratings and memory deficits that characterize these diagnoses.[17,18] Those interested in a more extensive set of regions within both the medial and lateral temporal lobes may find the extended scale of Galton and colleagues[19] useful.

Another viable option is the visual rating system to score the severity of medial temporal atrophy (VRS-MTA).[20] Using a 5-point scale, the VRS-MTA rates atrophy within a single coronal slice that intersects the mammillary bodies. Separate scores are calculated for the hippocampus, EC, and perirhinal cortex of each hemisphere. A library of reference images is available within the program, which facilitates the rating and improves reliability. In a large group of older adults (N = 224), Shen and colleagues[21] found that VRS-MTA scores could distinguish between older adults with no cognitive impairment, patients with MCI, and patients with AD. Receiver-operating characteristics analyses revealed that the VRS-MTA (area under the curve: .806–.819) more accurately distinguished healthy older adults from MCI patients than did hippocampal volumes (area under the curve: .725–.753). In addition, the VRS-MTA scores were slightly better related to clinical measures of memory functioning than were hippocampal volumes. In a separate study of 414 older adults, VRS-MTA–based ratings of even slight hippocampal and EC atrophy were associated with memory impairment.[22] The sensitivity of the VRS-MTA may be due to its measurement of the anterior hippocampus, which is where atrophy (especially the CA1 and subiculum subregions) is most prevalent in patients in MCI and also predictive of conversion to AD.[23] Thus, the ease of use, reliability, and apparent validity of the VRS-MTA all suggest it may hold promise for clinical practice.

Although the discussion here is limited to these 2 scales, other methods exist (see Soininen and colleagues[16] for a review), and may ultimately hold promise in the clinical assessment and diagnosis of those presenting with memory complaints.

Volumetric analyses

Volumetric analyses have long been used in AD research.[8] These techniques rely on the identification of hippocampal (or other structural) boundaries, and calculate the total volume by multiplying the number of voxels included within those boundaries by the voxel size. Thus, the accuracy of volumetric measurements is directly dependent on the quality (eg, lack of motion) and acquisition parameters of the scan. Several standardized and validated manual segmentation protocols exist for the hippocampus,[24,25] including some for data acquired at high field strength (eg, 7 T).[26] This approach can be exceedingly time consuming, especially at higher resolutions when more slices are acquired. Caution is warranted when selecting a manual approach because a recent study found up to a 2.5-fold difference in hippocampal volumes depending on the protocol used.[27] Differences also exist in protocols for measuring EC volume.[28] Semiautomated approaches that require the initial manual identification of key landmarks followed by an automated "filling" and volume calculation can save time, and have been sensitive to structural changes in those with MCI and AD.[29]

More recent efforts have created fully automated segmentation programs that are capable of calculating volumetrics with relatively little user input, which obviously increases the potential for their clinical adoption. FreeSurfer (http://surfer.nmr.mgh.harvard.edu) is a powerful and freely available neuroimaging analysis program that can provide whole-brain volumetrics as accurate as those resulting from manual segmentation, and which is also sensitive to the atrophy of medial temporal lobe that characterizes AD.[30] Despite these benefits, acquiring whole-brain volumetrics with FreeSurfer can be time consuming (about 24 hours per brain), and requires an experienced software user who must perform manual inspection of the data after several critical processing steps. An additional processing step provides volumetric data for 7 hippocampal subregions (CA1, CA2/3, CA4/dentate gyrus, presubiculum, subiculum, hippocampal fissure, and fimbria),[31] which may ultimately be informative when considering the etiology of memory impairment.[32] Despite the potential utility of these measures, there are no normative data nor are there thresholds that would support a diagnosis of MCI or AD; factors that limit the clinical utility of these values.

NeuroQuant (www.cortechslabs.com) is a commercially available program that originated from FreeSurfer, and has been approved by the Food and Drug Administration (FDA) for marketing as a medical device. It provides "whole-brain" volumetric analyses in about 15 minutes, although only a limited number of medial temporal regions are available (ie, amygdala, hippocampus, inferior lateral ventricles) and gross measurement of neocortical volumes is provided (eg, forebrain parenchyma; cortical gray matter). In the authors' experience, each analysis costs approximately $100, but physicians may be able to bill for this service and the associated interpretation using existing CPT codes. Given its origins in FreeSurfer, it is not surprising that the volumetric data from NeuroQuant have been validated against computer-aided manual segmentation programs, and that these values were sensitive to the changes demonstrated in AD.[33] In an initial pilot study of 17 older controls and 27 MCI patients, the authors found that each of the 3 medial temporal lobe values was significantly related to standardized memory test performance.[34] Especially relevant for clinical practice is an additional "Age-Related Atrophy Report" that compares hippocampal, inferior lateral ventricle, and lateral ventricle volumes for a given patient with age-matched individuals (which the report notes are for reference purposes only). Personal communication with staff at NeuroQuant (January 11, 2013 with Kora Marinkovic) indicated that normative data originate from the 200 control participants who took part in the Alzheimer's Disease Neuroimaging Initiative (ADNI; www.adni-info.org). These individuals were age 50 years or older, and all were cognitively intact. Although ADNI was a longitudinal study, only the initial scans from these individuals were used to calculate the normative data. The ease of use, clinical relevance of the measures provided, potential for billing, and use of normative data are all important advancements in this field that suggest NeuroQuant may be useful in clinical practice.

Measurement of White Matter Hyperintensities Using MRI

Although the primary focus of this review is on learning and memory, the authors deem it appropriate to discuss the cognitive ramifications of white matter hyperintensities (WMH) because these are often evident in patients with vascular risk factors such as hypertension, hyperlipidemia, and diabetes. WMH are common radiologic findings in the elderly,[35–37] and are often reported as "age-appropriate" or benign within radiologic reports. A substantial and growing body of evidence suggests that this is simply not the case, and that WMH can have significant effects on health and cognitive functioning. For example, a recent meta-analysis found that the presence of WMH was associated with increased risk of stroke, cognitive decline, dementia, and death.[38] With regard to cognitive functioning, WMH are consistently linked to deficient executive functioning and processing speed (see the meta-analysis by Gunning-Dixon and Raz[39]; see also Refs.[40–42]). Wright and colleagues[43] divided 656 older participants into quartiles based on WMH severity, which was measured using a semiautomated rating process. Participants with greatest WMH load (third and fourth quartiles) performed significantly worse on measures of fine motor speed, dexterity, and mental flexibility relative to participants in the first and second quartiles. Associations between both learning (ie, immediate recall) and memory (ie, delayed recall) and WMH severity have also been reported,[39,44] and suggest that WMH lesion load may contribute to the clinical presentation of memory deficits in MCI patients. In fact, MCI patients demonstrating both medial temporal atrophy and WMH experience greater and more widespread cognitive dysfunction and are more likely to convert to AD than are patients with either condition in isolation.[45] The relationship between MCI/AD and both WMH and microbleeds may arise from shared vascular risk factors and/or directly from AD pathology (eg, amyloid angiopathy) (see Hommet and colleagues[46] and Shoamanesh and colleagues[47] for reviews). Given such evidence, some have advocated that WMH should no longer be considered benign[48]; the authors generally agree, and provide a brief discussion of quantification methods that may facilitate the use of WMH severity within clinical practice (**Box 1**).

Visual rating scales

As with atrophy of the medial temporal lobe, WMH are most commonly evaluated using visual rating scales and volumetric analyses. These methods possess the same general limitations as the atrophy scales discussed earlier, although additional caution is needed when considering the locations used to assess WMH (eg, periventricular white matter, deep white matter, gray-white junction) (for full reviews see Scheltens and colleagues[49] or Kapeller and colleagues[50]). The Leukoaraiosis scale (LA)[51] assigns a score between 0 (no hyperintensities) and 4 (>75% hyperintensities) within 5 general regions within each hemisphere. These values are then combined to obtain a total score. Libon and colleagues[41] have used this scale extensively within the context of small vessel–based vascular dementia, and the authors previously reported differences in temporal-order memory in patients with high versus low LA scores.[52]

Box 1
Cognitive ramifications of white matter hyperintensities (WMH)

- WMH have been associated with increased risk of stroke, cognitive decline, dementia, and death

- WMH are associated with deficits in executive functioning and processing speed

- Some studies suggest that WMH lesion load may contribute to the clinical presentation of memory deficits in MCI

- MCI patients with both MTA and WMH have more severe and widespread cognitive deficits, and are more likely to convert to AD

- The relationship between MCI/AD and both WMH and microbleeds may arise from shared risk factors or directly from AD pathology

- Both visual rating scales and volumetric measurement of WMH can be performed and should be integrated within the clinical evaluation

Fazekas and colleagues'[53] scale uses a 4-point system to rate periventricular hyper-intensities (PVH) and deep white matter hyperintensities (DWMH) separately. This scale has been widely used, but only provides general information about the presence of WMH and little information regarding the distribution of WMH.[54] Scheltens and colleagues[54] extended the Fazekas scale to include subcortical hyperintesity ratings as well as the number, size, and location of the WMH. Although this scale provides a greater breadth of information, it is time consuming and applicable only to higher-quality MRI scans.

Volumetric analyses

Fully automated volumetric procedures have also been developed and seem promising, given the strong relationships with manual approaches.[55] Meier and colleagues[44] used an approach that first identified hyperintense areas (ie, ≥ 2.7 standard deviations above the mean intensity value of the entire image), then iteratively expanded the volume to adjacent voxels with intensity values within 5% of the seed region. These hyperintense volumes were also automatically localized within the brain (ie, frontal, parietal, temporal, occipital). Frontal and parietal WMH volumes were elevated in patients with MCI and further in AD relative to controls. Moreover, frontal WMH volumes were associated with greater memory impairment, again supporting the conclusion that these are not benign findings and should be considered within a clinical evaluation.

Computed Tomography

MRI can be cost prohibitive, contraindicated in some patients (eg, patients with metal implants or claustrophobia), or simply unavailable in some settings (eg, rural communities). Fortunately, computed tomography (CT) can also be used to assess structural changes. A recent study suggested that medial temporal lobe atrophy is best evaluated using the Jobst procedure, which uses a section plane 20° caudal to the orbito-meatal line through the posterior fossa and a slice thickness of 1.5 to 2 mm.[56,57] Structural thickness is calculated using calipers (for hard copies) or computer-based measurement programs for digital images. The minimum width of the temporal lobe is the primary variable of interest. Using this procedure, Frisoni and colleagues[58] found the width of the temporal horn to be a sensitive marker for AD. WMH visual rating scales have also been developed for CT (see Wahlund and colleagues[59] and Scheltens and colleagues[49]).

Positron Emission Tomography

Torosyan and Silverman[60] provide a clinically useful decision tree for determining the most appropriate type of positron emission tomography (PET) scan when confronted with a patient reporting or experiencing cognitive decline. The 2 main approaches and their relationship with cognitive functioning briefly discussed here.

Metabolic imaging

The ^{18}F-fluorodeoxyglucose (FDG) radioligand assesses glucose metabolism and has unquestionably added to our knowledge of brain-behavior relationships from a cognitive neuroscience perspective.[61] FDG-PET has several benefits in regard of the diagnosis and monitoring of those with AD, and has become a mainstay in the field as a result. Patients with AD demonstrate a characteristic metabolic reduction in both lateral (temporoparietal junction) and medial (posterior cingulate cortex, precuneus) posterior cortices.[60,62] In fact, the degree of hypometabolism in the midline regions is strongly related to disease severity,[63] and the inclusion of FDG-PET within a clinical evaluation can improve diagnostic accuracy (see Torosyan and Silverman[60] for a review). Caution is warranted, however, because neuropsychological testing and structural MRI more accurately predicted the clinical classification of patients with MCI and AD than did FDG-PET or cerebrospinal fluid measures, especially in those aged 75 years or older.[64] Regardless, a recent meta-analysis found that FDG-PET is 78.7% sensitive to, and 74% specific for, the conversion from MCI to AD over a 1- to 3-year period.[65] Important advancements have been made in attempts to standardize quantification methods, which are vital for reliable interpretation and diagnosis.[66] However, the direct assessment of learning and memory requires that scanning be paired with an active task, which is unlikely to occur within a clinical setting given the additional cost, time, and complexity of data acquisition and subsequent analysis. So although there is little doubt that FDG-PET can aid in the diagnostic process, clinically acquired data remain of limited benefit for assessing specific cognitive abilities.

β-amyloid imaging

The development of β-amyloid (Aβ) imaging techniques such as Pittsburgh Compound B (PIB)[67] and ^{18}F-AV-45[68] have revolutionized the in vivo detection of Aβ (but see Torosyan and Silverman[60] for a discussion of potential limitations). A meta-analysis revealed that PIB-PET appears to possess greater sensitivity (93.5%) but lower specificity (56.2%) when compared with FDG-PET in predicting conversion to AD.[65] PIB (and presumably AV-45) is also sensitive to Aβ deposition in asymptomatic elderly, with rates ranging from 19% to 83% depending on age (see Gelosa and Brooks[69] for a review). This property provides a unique opportunity to identify and track those at risk of eventually developing AD. The fact that the FDA recently approved AV-45 for the estimation of Aβ plaque density[70] will presumably result in its more widespread use in the near future. Although it is true that Aβ levels typically increase from "healthy" (ie, asymptomatic) elderly to those with a diagnosis of MCI and further to those with AD,[71] the relationship between Aβ load and cognition is unclear. For example, Villemagne and colleagues[71] observed a significant inverse relationship between episodic memory and posterior cingulate Aβ load in asymptomatic elderly, which seemingly supports this region's established role in memory functioning. However, an inverse relationship was also found between Aβ and episodic memory in every gray matter region examined, except the sensorimotor cortices, in MCI patients. This general relationship presumably reflects disease progression rather than a specific relationship between Aβ and memory abilities. Similarly, another recent study observed that Aβ load is poorly related to measures of cognitive functioning, including memory.[72] Such findings are consistent with histologic data of weaker associations between cognitive functioning and Aβ plaques than between cognitive functioning and neurofibrillary tangles (see Jack[62] for a more extensive review).

Neurofibrillary (tau) imaging

Experimental radioligands such as ^{18}F-FDDNP that bind to both Aβ and neurofibrillary tangles may be especially promising in the assessment of cognition.[73] Although considerably more work is needed in this area, some initial studies have shown that higher FDDNP binding was strongly correlated with overall cognitive functioning[74] and was predictive of cognitive decline at a 2-year follow-up.[75] As with Aβ imaging, however, evidence between binding in specific brain regions and the associated cognitive abilities is lacking at present. For example, increased global, frontal, and posterior cingulate FDDNP binding was significantly related to memory decline over a 2-year follow-up.[75] Such nonspecific relationships again warrant caution when attempting to infer cognitive functioning based on binding status alone.

In sum, the most clinically relevant and justified use of these emerging radiotracers is in the etiologic confirmation of symptomatic individuals and, potentially, in the prediction of conversion to a more severe disease state, but not in the direct measurement of cognitive functioning.

SECTION II: EXPERIMENTAL EVIDENCE OF NEUROPLASTIC CHANGE

Functional MRI (fMRI) has greatly informed our understanding of the neural mechanisms underlying cognitive changes across the spectrum from "healthy" aging to MCI to AD. Relative to PET, fMRI has many benefits including the widespread availability of MRI scanners, and its noninvasive nature (ie, fMRI does not require radioisotopes), high spatial resolution, and improved temporal resolution. Whereas FDG-PET is a direct measure of neuronal functioning, blood-oxygen level dependent (BOLD) fMRI is an indirect measure that relies on the measurement of deoxygenated hemoglobin. fMRI has typically only been used within research settings; however, it is gaining recognition as an effective tool in various clinical populations,[76,77] and some have advocated for its inclusion as a biomarker of AD.[78] As with FDG-PET, fMRI data can be acquired as the patient performs a cognitive task (ie, task-based) or during rest (ie, resting-state). This article focuses on task-based results because this approach reflects the use of specific cognitive abilities, whereas rest-state data are, at best, an indirect measure.

MCI-Associated Dysfunction

Meta-analyses of fMRI data have reinforced the importance of medial temporal lobe structures during learning and memory tasks in healthy individuals[79] and have shown hypoactivation of these structures in those with AD.[80] Whereas such results clearly demonstrate dysfunction in AD patients, an inconsistent pattern of hippocampal activation has emerged in MCI patients. For example, some studies have found hypoactivation[81–83] whereas others have reported hyperactivation relative to healthy controls.[84–86] Such findings led Dickerson and colleagues[78,87] to propose an inverse "U" relationship between activation and learning/memory functioning in MCI patients (see Dickerson and Sperling[87] or Sperling[78] for a review). This model posits that MCI patients who are less impaired (ie, those closer to the "normal" end of the spectrum) demonstrate an initial period of hippocampal hyperactivation that may reflect a compensatory mechanism and/or evidence of excitotoxicity. This stage is followed by a progressive decline in activation and associated memory functioning that eventually results in the hypoactive findings characteristic of AD patients.

The authors recently tested this inverse-U model in a study that required healthy older adults and patients with MCI to encode object-location associations.[88] Object-location associations are dependent on the hippocampus,[89] and the task was designed to be ecologically relevant by requiring participants to remember the location of objects within realistic-looking rooms. As expected, the healthy controls remembered significantly more novel associations than did the MCI patients. To avoid confounding attempted encoding with successful encoding, the fMRI analyses included only trials on which stimuli were successfully encoded (ie, subsequently remembered). At the group level, healthy controls demonstrated significantly greater hippocampal activation than did MCI patients. Hippocampal volume was comparable between the groups and, therefore, could not explain these differences. Because group-level analyses could obscure the individual differences that would result in an inverse U, the authors then examined the relationship between hippocampal β weights (ie, the regressor coefficients used to create the activation map) and measures of disease severity, defined here as hippocampal volume and the Total Score on the Repeatable Battery for Neuropsychological Status (RBANS). Whereas the healthy control group demonstrated significant relationships between right hippocampal activation and both volume and RBANS total score, there were no significant findings in the MCI group. Thus, these results failed to support the inverse-U model and suggest that key patient variables and/or methodological differences may account for the variable findings reported (see Hampstead and colleagues[88] for additional discussion).

Dysfunction is not limited to the hippocampus in MCI; rather, a growing body of evidence has revealed abnormal functioning in several interactive neocortical regions. A prefrontal-parietal network is known to mediate working memory (ie, the ability to mentally hold and manipulate information)[90,91] and to interact with the hippocampal memory system.[90] Functional neuroimaging studies have revealed increased prefrontal activity[91,92] as well as increased connectivity between the prefrontal cortex and hippocampal memory system during normal aging[93] that is often viewed as compensatory in nature.[94,95] Theoretically this may attenuate age-related reductions in hippocampal functioning.[96] Patients with MCI frequently demonstrate hypoactivation within this prefrontal-parietal network,[83,88,97] which suggests that the memory impairment in MCI is not solely due to dysfunction of the medial temporal lobe. In fact, the authors' recent study suggested that MCI patients may engage different cognitive mechanisms while attempting to learn new information, because performance was significantly related to activation within the primary motor and somatosensory cortices in MCI patients in comparison with the expected prefrontal-parietal network in healthy controls.[88] Thus, a key question is whether interventions designed to improve learning and memory can reengage the "normal" brain regions and/or recruit additional areas in a compensatory manner in patients with MCI.

Evidence of Neuroplasticity Following Treatment

Many of the techniques discussed herein hold promise in predicting and measuring the effects of both pharmacologic and nonpharmacologic interventions. In fact, several groups have used both structural and functional neuroimaging to examine neuroplastic change following cognitive rehabilitation. Cognitive rehabilitation of memory is considered a practice standard for some patient populations with static insults,[98] and comprehensive reviews[99,100] and a meta-analysis[101] have surmised that it is of benefit to those with MCI. With regard to structural imaging, hippocampal volumes predicted treatment-based improvement in older adults with subjective memory complaints.[102] Similarly, the authors' recent randomized controlled trial found that the volume of the inferior lateral ventricles was inversely related to memory test improvement after cognitive rehabilitation in patients with MCI.[103] Of note, no relationship existed in the control group who was matched for the number of stimulus exposures. Such results suggest that the same measures of atrophy that aid the diagnostic process may ultimately help inform treatment planning.

fMRI has been used to examine the neuroplastic effects of cognitive rehabilitation, especially mnemonic strategies, involving techniques such as semantic organization, semantic elaboration, and mental imagery. Mnemonic-strategy training has increased activation within prefrontal and parietal regions[104–106] as well as the hippocampus[107] in healthy young individuals. The authors previously reported that mnemonic-strategy training not only improved learning and memory of face-name associations[108] but also resulted in increased activation within a distributed network that involved the prefrontal and parietal cortices (among other regions).[81] In addition, effective connectivity analyses revealed increased interaction between many of these regions, supporting the possibility that these changes reflect the functional reorganization of cognitive processing. Other groups have documented both restorative and compensatory changes in prefrontal, parietal, and temporal cortices following a memory rehabilitation program in patients with MCI.[109] The obvious hope is that increased activation within these neocortical regions facilitates hippocampal functioning. In fact, the authors' randomized controlled trial clearly demonstrated increased hippocampal activity in the mnemonic-strategy–trained group of MCI patients, whereas the matched-exposure group showed no such changes.[110] Together, these fMRI results provide evidence for treatment-induced neuroplasticity in those with MCI, and may ultimately aid in the selective targeting of brain regions that would mitigate memory dysfunction.

SUMMARY

The general field of aging and dementia (including Geriatric Medicine, Neurology, and Neuropsychology) has benefited greatly from the synergism that exists between clinical and research settings. The literature reviewed herein indicates that structural neuroimaging–based measures of medial temporal lobe atrophy often correspond to objective memory impairment, may help predict conversion to dementia, and may help in developing a treatment plan for those with MCI. Although common in an elderly population WMH should not be considered benign, because they have been associated with executive and memory dysfunction, and the combination of atrophy and WMH suggests more rapid progression to AD. Therefore, clinical practice could greatly benefit from the inclusion of standardized ratings of atrophy and WMH, although care is needed when selecting the exact measurement technique(s). PET (both metabolic and Aβ) can also meaningfully inform the diagnostic process, but clinically acquired data are likely to be of limited use when considering specific cognitive abilities. Finally, fMRI has greatly informed our understanding of the widespread changes in cognitive processing that occur in those with MCI, and has also provided evidence of preserved neuroplasticity in this population. These and future findings will be critical as clinical researchers confront the next great challenge in aging and dementia: the treatment of those at various points along the AD spectrum.

REFERENCES

1. Rosen HJ, Gorno-Tempeni ML, Goldman WP, et al. Patterns of brain atrophy in frontotemporal dementia and semantic dementia. Neurology 2002;58:198–208.
2. Ashford JW, Salehi A, Furst A, et al. Imaging the Alzheimer brain. J Alzheimers Dis 2011;26:1–27.
3. Jack CR Jr, Knopman DS, Jagust WJ, et al. Hypothetical model of dynamic biomarkers of the Alzheimer's pathological cascade. Lancet 2010;9:119–28.
4. Albert MS, Dekosky ST, Dickson D, et al. The diagnosis of mild cognitive impairment due to Alzheimer's disease: recommendations from the National Institute on Aging-Alzheimer's Association workgroups on diagnostic guidelines for Alzheimer's disease. Alzheimers Dement 2011;7:270–9.
5. Jacova C, Kertesz A, Blair M, et al. Neuropsychological testing and assessment for dementia. Alzheimers Dement 2007;3:299–317.
6. Anstey KJ, Maller JJ. The role of volumetric MRI in understanding mild cognitive impairment and similar classifications. Aging Ment Health 2003;7:2238–50.
7. De Leon MJ, George AE, Stylopoulos LA, et al. Early marker for Alzheimer's disease: the atrophic hippocampus. Lancet 1989;2:672–3.
8. Jack CR Jr, Petersen RC, Xu YC, et al. Medial temporal atrophy on MRI in normal aging and very mild Alzheimer's disease. Neurology 1997;49:786–94.

9. Schroeter ML, Stein T, Maslowski N, et al. Neural correlates of Alzheimer's disease and mild cognitive impairment: a systematic and quantitative meta-analysis involving 1351 patients. Neuroimage 2009;47:1196–206.

10. Raz N, Rodrigue KM. Differential aging of the brain: patterns, cognitive correlates and modifiers. Neurosci Biobehav Rev 2006;30:730–48.

11. Petersen RC, Parisi JE, Dickson DW, et al. Neuropathologic features of amnestic mild cognitive impairment. Arch Neurol 2006;63:665–72.

12. Chetelat G, Baron J. Early diagnosis of Alzheimer's disease: contribution of structural neuroimaging. Neuroimage 2003;18:525–41.

13. Gold JJ, Squire LR. Quantifying medial temporal lobe damage in memory-impaired patients. Hippocampus 2005;15:79–85.

14. Scarmeas N, Yaakov S. Cognitive reserve: implications for diagnosis and prevention of Alzheimer's disease. Curr Neurol Neurosci Rep 2004;4:374–80.

15. Scheltens P, Leys D, Barkhof F, et al. Atrophy of medial temporal lobes on MRI in "probable" Alzheimer's disease and normal ageing: diagnostic value and neuropsychological correlates. J Neurol Neurosurg Psychiatr 1992;55: 967–72.

16. Soininen H, Yawu L, Rueckert D, et al. Hippocampal atrophy in Alzheimer's disease. Neurodegener Dis Manag 2012;2:197–209.

17. Westman E, Cavallin L, Muehlboeck JS, et al. Sensitivity and specificity of medial temporal lobe visual ratings and multivariate regional MRI classification in Alzheimer's disease. PLoS One 2011;6:e22506.

18. Shim YS, Young CY, Duk LN, et al. Effects of medial temporal atrophy and white matter hyperintensities on the cognitive functions in patients with Alzheimer's disease. Eur Neurol 2011;66:75–82.

19. Galton CJ, Gomez-Anson B, Antoun N, et al. Temporal lobe rating scale: application to Alzheimer's disease and frontotemporal dementia. J Neurol Neurosurg Psychiatr 2001;70:165–73.

20. Duara R, Loewenstein DA, Potter E, et al. Medial temporal lobe atrophy on MRI scans and the diagnosis of Alzheimer disease. Neurology 2008;71:1986–92.

21. Shen Q, Loewenstein DA, Potter E, et al. Volumetric and visual rating of MRI scans in the diagnosis of amnestic MCI and Alzheimer's disease. Alzheimers Dement 2011;7:1–17.

22. Varon D, Loewenstein DA, Potter E, et al. Minimal atrophy of the entorhinal cortex and hippocampus: progression of cognitive impairment. Dement Geriatr Cogn Disord 2011;31:276–83.

23. Devanand DP, Bansal R, Liu J, et al. MRI hippocampal and entorhinal cortex mapping in predicting conversion to Alzheimer's disease. Neuroimage 2012; 60:1622–9.

24. Malykhin NV, Bouchard TP, Ogilvie CJ, et al. Three-dimensional volumetric analysis and reconstruction of amygdala and hippocampal head, body, and tail. Psychiatry Res 2007;155:155–65.

25. Pruessner JC, Li LM, Serles W, et al. Volumetry of hippocampus and amygdala with high-resolution MRI and three-dimensional analysis software: minimizing the discrepancies between laboratories. Cereb Cortex 2000;10:433–42.

26. Wisse LE, Gerritsen L, Zwanenburg JJ, et al. Subfields of the hippocampal formation at 7T MRI: In vivo volumetric assessment. Neuroimage 2012;61: 1043–9.

27. Boccardi M, Ganzola R, Bocchetta M, et al. Survey of protocols for the manual segmentation of the hippocampus: preparatory steps towards a joint EADC-ADNI harmonized protocol. J Alzheimers Dis 2011;26:61–75.

28. Price CC, Wood MF, Leonard CM, et al. Entorhinal cortex volume in older adults: reliability and validity considerations for three published measurement protocols. J Int Neuropsychol Soc 2010;16:846–55.

29. Nestor SM, Rupsingh R, Borrie M, et al. Ventricular enlargement as a possible measure of Alzheimer's disease progression validated using the Alzheimer's disease neuroimaging initiative database. Brain 2008;131:2443–54.

30. Fischl B, Salat DH, Busa E, et al. Whole brain segmentation: automated labeling of neuroanatomical structures in the human brain. Neuron 2002;33:341–55.

31. Van Leemput K, Bakkour A, Benner T, et al. Automated segmentation of hippocampal subfields from ultra-high resolution in vivo MRI. Hippocampus 2009;19: 549–57.

32. Small SA, Schobel SA, Buxton RB, et al. A pathophysiological framework of hippocampal dysfunction in ageing and disease. Nat Rev Neurosci 2011;12:585–601.

33. Brewer JB, Magda S, Airriess C, et al. Fully automated quantification of regional brain volumes for improved detection of focal atrophy in Alzheimer's disease. AJNR Am J Neuroradiol 2009;30:578–80.

34. Tedjopranoto J, Hampstead BM. Assessing the relationship between RBANS normative data and medial temporal volumetrics in mild cognitive impairment. J Int Neuropsychol Soc 2011;S1:117.

35. Breteler MM, van Swieten JC, Bots ML, et al. Cerebral white matter lesions, vascular risk factors, and cognitive function in a population-based study: the Rotterdam Study. Neurology 1994;44:1246–52.

36. Lindgren AI, Roijer A, Rudling O, et al. Cerebral lesions on magnetic resonance imaging, heart disease, and vascular risk factors in subjects without stroke. A population-based study. Stroke 1994;25:929–34.

37. Manolio TA, Kronmal RA, Burke GL, et al. Magnetic resonance abnormalities and cardiovascular disease in older adults. The Cardiovascular Health Study. Stroke 1994;25:318–27.

38. Debette S, Markus HS. The clinical importance of white matter hyperintensities on brain magnetic resonance imaging: systematic review and meta-analysis. BMJ 2010;341:c3666.

39. Gunning-Dixon FM, Raz N. The cognitive correlates of white matter abnormalities in normal aging: a quantitative review. Neuropsychology 2000;14: 224–32.

40. Delano-Wood L, Bondi MW, Sacco J, et al. Heterogeneity in mild cognitive impairment: differences in neuropsychological and associated white mater lesion pathology. J Int Neuropsychol Soc 2009;15:906–14.

41. Libon DJ, Price CC, Giovannetti T, et al. Linking MRI hyperintensities with patterns of neuropsychological impairment—evidence for a threshold effect. Stroke 2008;39:806–13.

42. Romos-Estebanez C, Moral-Arce I, Gonzalez-Mandly A, et al. Vascular cognitive impairment in small vessel disease: clinical and neuropsychological features of lacunar state and Binswanger's disease. Age Ageing 2011;40:175–80.

43. Wright CB, Festa JR, Paik MC, et al. White matter hyperintensities and subclinical infarction: associations with psychomotor speed and cognitive flexibility. Stroke 2008;39:800–5.

44. Meier IB, Manly JJ, Provenzano FA, et al. White matter predictors of cognitive functioning in older adults. J Int Neuropsychol Soc 2012;18:414–27.

45. Rossi R, Geroldi C, Bresciani L, et al. Clinical and neuropsychological features associated with structural imaging patterns in patients with mild cognitive impairment. Dement Geriatr Cogn Disord 2007;23:175–83.

46. Hommet C, Mondon K, Constans T, et al. Review of cerebral microangiopathy and Alzheimer's disease: relation between white matter hyperintensities and microbleeds. Dement Geriatr Cogn Disord 2011;32:367–78.

47. Shoamanesh A, Kwok CS, Benavente O. Cerebral microbleeds: histopathological correlation of neuroimaging. Cerebrovasc Dis 2011;32:528–34.

48. Kuo H, Lipsitz LA. Cerebral white matter changes and geriatric syndromes: is there a link? J Gerontol B Psychol Sci Soc Sci 2004;59A:818–26.

49. Scheltens P, Erkinjunti T, Didier L, et al. White matter changes on CT and MRI: an overview of visual rating scales. Eur Neurol 1998;39:80–9.

50. Kapeller P, Barber R, Vermeulen RJ, et al. Visual rating of age-related white matter changes on magnetic resonance imaging: scale comparison, interrater agreement, and correlations with quantitative measurements. Stroke 2003;34: 441–5.

51. Junque C, Pujol J, Vendrell P, et al. Leuko-araiosis on magnetic resonance imaging and speed of mental processing. Arch Neurol 1990;47:151–6.

52. Hampstead BM, Libon DJ, Moetler ST, et al. Temporal order memory differences in Alzheimer's disease and vascular dementia. J Clin Exp Neuropsychol 2010; 32:645–54.

53. Fazekas F, Chawluk JB, Alavi A, et al. MR signal abnormalities as 1.5 T in Alzheimer's dementia and normal aging. AJR Am J Roentgenol 1987;149:351–6.

54. Scheltens P, Barkhof D, Leys JP, et al. A semiquantitative rating scale for the assessment of signal hyperintensities on magnetic resonance imaging. J Neurol Sci 1993;114:7–12.

55. Wu M, Rosano C, Butlers M, et al. A fully automated method for quantifying and localizing white matter hyperintensities on MR images. Psychiatry Res 2006; 148:133–42.

56. Jobst KA, Smith AD, Szatmari M, et al. Detection in life of confirmed Alzheimer's disease using a simple measurement of medial temporal lobe atrophy by computed tomography. Lancet 1992;340:1179–83.

57. Pasi M, Poggesi A, Pantoni L. The use of CT in dementia. Int Psychogeriatr 2011;23:S6–12.

58. Frisoni GB, Geroldi C, Beltramello A, et al. Radial width of the temporal horn: a sensitive measure in Alzheimer disease. AJNR Am J Neuroradiol 2002;23:35–47.

59. Wahlund LO, Barkhof F, Fazekas F, et al. A new rating scale for age-related white matter changes applicable to MRI and CT. Stroke 2001;32:1318–22.

60. Torosyan N, Silverman DH. Neuronuclear imaging in the evaluation of dementia and mild decline in cognition. Semin Nucl Med 2012;42:415–22.

61. Cabeza R, Nyberg L. Imaging cognition II: an empirical review of 275 PET and fMRI studies. J Cogn Neurosci 2000;12:1–47.

62. Jack CR. Alzheimer disease: new concepts on its neurobiology and the clinical role imaging will play. Radiology 2012;263:344–61.

63. Langbaum JB, Chen K, Lee W, et al. Categorical and correlational analyses of baseline fluorodeoxyglucose positron emission tomography images from the Alzheimer's Disease Neuroimaging Initiative (ADNI). Neuroimage 2009;45: 1107–16.

64. Schmand B, Eikelenboom P, van Gool WA. Value of neuropsychological tests, neuroimaging, and biomarkers for diagnosing Alzheimer's disease in younger and older age cohorts. J Am Geriatr Soc 2011;59:1705–10.

65. Zhang S, Han D, Tan X, et al. Diagnostic accuracy of ^{18}F-FDG and ^{11}C-PIB PET for prediction of short-term conversion to Alzheimer's disease in subjects with mild cognitive impairment. Int J Clin Pract 2012;66:185–98.

66. Caroli A, Prestia A, Chen K, et al. Summary metrics to assess Alzheimer disease related hypometabolic pattern with F-18-FDG PET: head to head comparison. J Nucl Med 2012;53:592–600.
67. Klunk WE, Engler H, Nordberg A, et al. Imaging brain amyloid in Alzheimer's disease with Pittsburgh Compound-B. Ann Neurol 2004;55:306–19.
68. Wong DF, Rosenberg PB, Zhou Y, et al. In vivo imaging of amyloid deposition in Alzheimer disease using the radioligand 18F-AV-45 (florbetapir). J Nucl Med 2010;51:913–20.
69. Gelosa G, Brooks DJ. The prognostic value of amyloid imaging. Eur J Nucl Med Mol Imaging 2012;39:1207–19.
70. Romano M, Buratti E. Florbetapir F18 for brain imaging of β-amyloid plaques. Drugs Today (Barc) 2013;49(3):181–93.
71. Villemagne VL, Pike KE, Chetelat G, et al. Longitudinal assessment of Aβ and cognition in aging and Alzheimer disease. Ann Neurol 2011;69:181–92.
72. Furst AJ, Rabinovici GD, Rostomian AH, et al. Cognition, glucose metabolism and amyloid burden in Alzheimer's disease. Neurobiol Aging 2012;33:215–25.
73. Shin J, Kepe V, Barrio JR, et al. The merits of FDDNP-PET imaging in Alzheimer's disease. J Alzheimers Dis 2011;26:135–45.
74. Braskie MN, Klunder AD, Hayashi KM, et al. Plaque and tangle imaging and cognition in normal aging and Alzheimer's disease. Neurobiol Aging 2010;31:1669–78.
75. Small GW, Siddarth P, Kepe V, et al. Prediction of cognitive decline by positron emission tomography of brain amyloid and tau. Arch Neurol 2012;69:215–22.
76. Beers CA, Federico P. Functional MRI applications in epilepsy surgery. Can J Neurol Sci 2012;39:271–85.
77. Zaca D, Nickerson JP, Delb G, et al. Effectiveness of four different clinical fMRI paradigms for preoperative regional determination of language lateralization in patients with brain tumors. Neuroradiology 2012;54:1015–25.
78. Sperling RA. The potential of functional MRI as a biomarker in early Alzheimer's disease. Neurobiol Aging 2011;32:S37–43.
79. Spaniol J, Davidson PS, Kim AS, et al. Event-related fMRI studies of episodic encoding and retrieval: meta-analyses using activation likelihood estimation. Neuropsychologia 2009;47:1765–79.
80. Schwindt GC, Black SE. Functional imaging studies of episodic memory in Alzheimer's disease: a quantitative meta-analysis. Neuroimage 2009;45:181–90.
81. Hampstead BM, Stringer AY, Stilla RF, et al. Activation and effective connectivity changes following explicit-memory training for face-name pairs in patients with MCI: a pilot study. Neurorehabil Neural Repair 2011;25:210–22.
82. Johnson SC, Saykin AJ, Baxter LC, et al. The relationship between fMRI activation and cerebral atrophy: comparison of normal aging and Alzheimer's disease. Neuroimage 2004;11:179–87.
83. Machulda MM, Senjem ML, Weigand SD, et al. Functional magnetic resonance imaging changes in amnestic and nonamnestic mild cognitive impairment during encoding and recognition tasks. J Int Neuropsychol Soc 2009;15:372–82.
84. Dickerson BC, Salat DH, Greve DN, et al. Increased hippocampal activation in mild cognitive impairment compared to normal aging and AD. Neurology 2005;65:404–11.
85. Hamalainen A, Pihlajamaki M, Tanila H, et al. Increased fMRI responses during encoding in mild cognitive impairment. Neurobiol Aging 2007;28:1809–903.

86. Kircher TT, Wels S, Freymann K, et al. Hippocampal activation in patients with mild cognitive impairment is necessary for successful memory encoding. J Neurol Neurosurg Psychiatr 2007;78:812–8.

87. Dickerson BC, Sperling RA. Functional abnormalities of the medial temporal lobe memory system in mild cognitive impairment and Alzheimer's disease: insights from functional MRI studies. Neuropsychologia 2008;46:1624–35.

88. Hampstead BM, Stringer AY, Stilla RF, et al. Where did I put that? Patients with aMCI demonstrate widespread reductions in activity. Neuropsychologia 2011; 49:2349–61.

89. Postma A, Kessels RP, van Asselen M. How the brain remembers and forgets where things are: the neurocognition of object-location memory. Neurosci Biobehav Rev 2008;32:1339–45.

90. Baddeley A. Working memory: looking back and looking forward. Nat Rev Neurosci 2003;4:829–39.

91. Cabeza R. Hemispheric asymmetry reduction in older adults: the HAROLD model. Psychol Aging 2002;17:85–100.

92. Cabeza R, Anderson ND, Locantore JK, et al. Aging gracefully: compensatory brain activity in high-performing older adults. Neuroimage 2002;17: 1394–402.

93. Dennis NA, Hayes SM, Prince SE, et al. Effects of aging on the neural correlates of successful item and source memory encoding. J Exp Psychol Learn Mem Cogn 2008;34:791–808.

94. Park DC, Reuter-Lorenz P. The adaptive brain: aging and neurocognitive scaffolding. Annu Rev Psychol 2009;60:173–96.

95. Davis SW, Dennis NA, Daselaar SM, et al. Que PASA? the posterior-anterior shift in aging. Cereb Cortex 2008;18:1201–9.

96. Brickman AM, Stern Y, Small SA. Hippocampal subregions differentially associate with standardized memory tests. Hippocampus 2011;21:923–8.

97. Mandzia JL, McAndrews MP, Grady CL, et al. Neural correlates of incidental memory in MCI. Neurobiol Aging 2009;30:717–30.

98. Cicerone KD, Langenbahn DM, Braden C, et al. Evidence-based cognitive rehabilitation: updated review of the literature from 2003 through 2008. Arch Phys Med Rehabil 2011;92:519–30.

99. Jean L, Bergeron M, Thivierge S, et al. Cognitive intervention programs for individuals with mild cognitive impairment: systematic review of the literature. Am J Geriatr Psychiatry 2010;18:281–96.

100. Simon SS, Yokomizo JE, Bottino CM. Cognitive intervention in amnestic mild cognitive impairment: a systematic review. Neurosci Biobehav Rev 2012;36: 1163–78.

101. Li H, Li J, Li N, et al. Cognitive intervention for persons with MCI: a meta-analysis. Ageing Res Rev 2011;10:285–96.

102. Engvig A, Fjell AM, Westlye LT, et al. Hippocampal subfield volumes correlate with memory training benefit in subjective memory impairment. Neuroimage 2012;61:188–94.

103. Hampstead BM, Sathian K, Phillips PA, et al. Mnemonic strategy training improves memory for object location associations in both healthy elderly and patients with aMCI. Neuropsychology 2012;26:385–99.

104. Kondo Y, Suzuki M, Mugikura S, et al. Changes in brain activation associated with use of a memory strategy: a functional MRI study. Neuroimage 2005;24:1154–63.

105. Miotto EC, Savage CR, Evans JJ, et al. Bilateral activation of PFC after strategic semantic cognitive training. Hum Brain Mapp 2006;27:288–95.

106. Savage CR, Deckersbach T, Heckers S, et al. Prefrontal regions supporting spontaneous and directed application of verbal learning strategies—evidence from PET. Brain 2001;124:219–31.
107. Nyberg L, Sandblam J, Jones S, et al. Neural correlates of training-related memory improvement. Proc Natl Acad Sci U S A 2003;100:13728–33.
108. Hampstead BM, Sathian K, Moore AB, et al. Explicit memory training leads to improved memory for face-name pairs in patients with mild cognitive impairment: results of a pilot investigation. J Int Neuropsychol Soc 2008;14:883–9.
109. Belleville S, Clement F, Mellah S, et al. Training-related brain plasticity in subjects at risk of developing Alzheimer's disease. Brain 2011;134:1623–34.
110. Hampstead BM, Stringer AY, Stilla RF, et al. Mnemonic strategy training partially restores hippocampal activity in patients with mild cognitive impairment. Hippocampus 2012;22:1652–8.

Current Management Decisions in Mild Cognitive Impairment

Benjamin A. Bensadon, EdM, PhD[a],*,
Germaine L. Odenheimer, MD[b]

KEYWORDS

- Impairment • MCI • Dementia • Cognition • Memory

KEY POINTS

- Mild cognitive impairment (MCI) is a clinical concept characterized by heterogeneous cause, clinical course, and research literature.
- Reversible causes of MCI can be targeted directly.
- There are no approved medications to prevent or treat MCI symptoms or progression.
- Controlling vascular risk factors may be considered an important aspect of MCI management.
- Clinicians should collaboratively partner with patients and caregivers to optimally manage the implications of diagnostic and prognostic uncertainty; emphasizing functional independence and quality of life.

INTRODUCTION

Management of mild cognitive impairment (MCI) is anything but straightforward. First described in the late 1980s and further characterized in the early 1990s,[1–6] in the ensuing decades, myriad terms, definitions, and scoring systems have been introduced and refined in an attempt to accurately operationalize, measure, classify, quantify, and categorize this clinical phenomenon, distinguishing it as more severe than normative age-related memory and cognitive problems, and milder than dementia. Careful review of the extant literature reveals a persistent lack of consensus not only in terms of how best to manage MCI, but relatedly, what it is and how it should be defined. As shown throughout this article, establishing best practice guidelines is thus confounded because MCI encapsulates a heterogeneous patient population and a body of literature plagued by inconsistent research methodology.

[a] Donald W. Reynolds Department of Geriatric Medicine, University of Oklahoma Health Sciences Center, 1122 NE 13th Street, ORB 1200, Oklahoma City, OK 73117, USA; [b] Donald W. Reynolds Department of Geriatric Medicine, University of Oklahoma Health Sciences Center, and Oklahoma City VA Medical Center, Oklahoma City, OK, USA
* Corresponding author.
E-mail address: Benjamin.bensadon@gmail.com

Clin Geriatr Med 29 (2013) 847–871
http://dx.doi.org/10.1016/j.cger.2013.07.008
0749-0690/13/$ – see front matter © 2013 Elsevier Inc. All rights reserved.

MCI is often conceptualized as a prodromal, preclinical, or subclinical stage of dementia, particularly Alzheimer disease (AD).[7] Corroborating this view has been evidence suggesting annual conversion rates from MCI to AD of approximately 10% to 15% per year compared with 1% to 2% among nonimpaired elderly.[6,8,9] MCI affects both sexes; however, unlike AD prevalence rates, some data suggest higher MCI prevalence among men after controlling for chronologic age.[10] In part because of the diagnostic heterogeneity alluded to earlier, rates of dementia progression have been variable,[11,12] but studies with longer follow-up periods (ie, 6–9 years) have shown greater conversion (80%–100%).[7,13] One study of 3063 community-dwellers diagnosed with MCI at baseline yielded different conversion rates depending on diagnostic criteria (functional vs cognitive/neuropsychological) used.[14]

Adding complexity to this picture is the fact that progression is not inevitable, and evidence for MCI-related deficits remaining stable or even reversing is not insignificant.[11,15,16] One recent prospective study of 1517 participants (≥65 years old)[17] found that almost twice as many individuals originally diagnosed with MCI reverted to normal functioning (n = 61) as those who converted to dementia (n = 35) at 2-year follow-up. Evidence of such reversibility has led some to suggest MCI may be more accurately considered a dementia risk factor.[18] Such conflicting evidence seems the rule rather than the exception, and although MCI continues to garner attention from the medical and scientific communities, complexity endures.

In practice, the first indication that something is wrong, cognitively, is either subjective memory complaint, or, when previously managed, chronic, comorbid conditions become increasingly difficult to control (eg, diabetes mellitus). When this information is presented to the clinician, a structured, thorough history taking is often recommended.[19] This history includes screening for depression, a condition frequently linked to memory complaint[20] and a possibly reversible cause of MCI. Reliance on subjective memory reports, be they from patients or informants, is controversial, given the conflicting evidence of their reliability and validity.[21] Furthermore, neurodegenerative processes likely begin long before initial complaints occur.[22,23] Therefore, clinicians' ability to accurately detect such patterns relies on careful historical comparison with previous levels of cognitive function, which, initially, can be provided only by informants or patients themselves.

Standard assessment involves comparison of cognitive performance on screening tools such as the Mini-Mental State Examination (MMSE),[24] and neuropsychological test performance to age-based and education-based normative data. For MCI, some have set a cutoff of 1 standard deviation lower than these means, whereas others have used a more stringent cutoff of 1.5. Although inconsistent cutoffs may be problematic, objective baseline assessment at only 1 time point is insufficient when considering possible neurodegenerative processes. Some have criticized an overreliance on testing and underutilization of informants.[7]

Heterogeneity

Compounding the inherent clinical challenges of cognitive impairment are inconsistencies of MCI operationalization and nosology, which have led to disparities in reported prevalence and incidence estimates both between and even within definitions.[25] Most recently, members of the National Institute on Aging-Alzheimer's Association Workgroup have proposed a new term, "MCI due to AD."[26] Although methodological and diagnostic heterogeneity must be rectified, there are several broad, widely accepted conceptual criteria for MCI that guide this article.[6,27] These criteria are:

- Subjectively reported memory complaints (by informant or patient)

- Objectively confirmed memory impairment for age and education level
- Preserved and generally intact cognitive function and activities of daily living (ADL)

Initially characterized in relation to eventual AD, these criteria reveal a decided memory focus. More recently, these criteria were revised to allow for other impaired cognitive domains, independent of memory. This revision resulted in 4 MCI subtypes depending on how many cognitive domains are affected (ie, single vs multiple) and whether memory is among them (ie, amnestic vs nonamnestic):

- MCI-amnestic, single domain (MCI-a)
- MCI-nonamnestic, single domain (MCI-na)
- MCI-amnestic, multiple domain (MCI-a-md)
- MCI-nonamnestic, multiple domain (MCI-na-md)

Although many agree with these criteria and core characteristics, challenges to optimal treatment recommendations remain. Adequate management of any illness benefits from clear understanding of the disease state (ie, pathophysiology) itself. As this article shows, this understanding has not yet been established for MCI.[28] In geriatric primary care, cognitive screening with asymptomatic individuals is not routine practice, and according to an evidence-based report of the American Academy of Neurology, it should not be.[13] Even when indicated, screening tools lack a gold standard of measurement,[29] performance score cutoffs for MCI designation differ, and although specific biomarkers show promise,[30] like those for AD, their evidence is mixed and remains speculative.[31–34] As mentioned earlier, even with accurate diagnostic classification, the subsequent course of MCI is often unstable, with reversion to normal cognitive function (without intervention) not uncommon.[11,12] More specifically, some have reported reversal rates of 33% to 56% over 1 to 2.5 years,[9,15,35,36] 5% to 20% over 3 to 3.5 years,[37–41] and 1 study reported MCI reversal in nearly half the sample (42%) over a 5-year time frame.[42] Such heterogeneity has led some to question its legitimacy as a clinical entity, concluding that without further refinement, devising specific treatment may be premature.[43]

Although such complexity makes effective clinical management a daunting task, well-documented increases in life expectancy and growing incidence of neurodegenerative illness, for which age is the number 1 risk factor, underscore its urgent and timely nature. Still a comparatively new concept, MCI has not been examined as extensively as dementia. This situation may be changing, however, because cognitive impairment is increasingly diagnosed, although it may or may not convert to dementia. Some large population-based studies have estimated that prevalence rates of cognitive impairment with no dementia (CIND) are more than double those of dementia.[44,45]

Amidst these challenges, this article serves as a clinical resource for management decisions based on reviews of the extant scientific literature. Given the nascent level of understanding of MCI as a unique disease state, our focus is on considerations and suggestions (ie, ethical, functional, technological, behavioral) as opposed to strict guidelines, which would not be sufficiently supported by the evidence. Our primary goal is to aid clinicians in maximizing their ability to effectively manage this diverse, rapidly increasing patient population.

Most notable in reviewing the extant literature, beyond the complexity, is a paucity of treatment options. Given the rationale outlined earlier, to some degree, the disproportionate emphasis on diagnostics is reasonable. However, the degree to which resources (human and financial) have targeted evaluation and diagnosis, to the exclusion of management, is problematic. Most MCI literature has focused on theorizing mechanisms of action, identifying biomarkers, and refining evaluation, screening, and assessment techniques, with scant attention dedicated to treatment.[46]

Dementia Staging

MCI is increasingly considered the earliest stage of dementia. The Clinical Dementia Rating (CDR)[47,48] and the Global Deterioration Scale (GDS)[49] are the most well-known instruments used to stage patients' progress along a dementia continuum. Assessment with these tools is primarily based on functional and cognitive status (ADL/neuropsychological testing).

The CDR is a clinically based, semistructured interview, which rates impairment level in 6 cognitive domains: memory, orientation, judgment/problem solving, community affairs, home and hobbies, and personal care. Scores are determined on a 5-point Likert scale for each domain, in which 0, 1, 2, or 3 correspond to dementia severity levels of none, early, moderate, and severe. Original longitudinal data included many patients who showed evidence of cognitive impairment that made AD suspected but insufficient for a definite diagnosis (ie, early dementia). Therefore, the scoring system was refined such that these individuals were given a CDR score of 0.5, which represented suspected or questionable dementia, now frequently referred to as MCI. Over 7 years, 11 of the 16 study participants staged at 0.5 progressed to AD or another CDR stage at which dementia was evident.[1]

Similarly, the GDS enumerates 7 stages. In practice, although patients and families may express a desire for specific stage information (early/middle/late or mild/moderate/severe), articulating the differences between stages can be cumbersome. Stages 2 and 3 and CDR 0.5 are considered analogous to MCI.[27] Both instruments are largely based on typical AD trajectories, thus related disorders such as normal pressure hydrocephalus, frontal dementias, vascular dementias (VaDs), and dementia with Lewy bodies, do not fit neatly into these staging models. Generally, they are better suited for clinical research and specialty settings (eg, dementia clinics) rather than primary care.

Vascular Risk Factors

Disentangling the role of vascular risk factors (VRF) in MCI and AD is complex, and their overlapping features and frequent coexistence are well established.[50] VaD, previously labeled multiinfarct dementia, is the second most common subtype behind AD. Early neuropathologic descriptions of dementia of vascular origin date back to the late 1800s.[51] More than a century later, despite significant progress, diagnostic challenges continue, definitions vary, and the relationship between vascular disease and dementia remains shrouded in controversy.[52] Vascular diseases such as hypercholesterolemia and hypertension may confer increased risk for MCI[8,53] and subsequent conversion to AD.[54,55]

One of the most well-known studies to shed light on the relationship of VRF and dementia was the nun study, begun in 1986.[56] Prospective data collection continues from an original sample of 678 American Roman Catholic nuns. Among an array of relevant published findings, Snowdon and colleagues[57] examined a subsample of 102 participants (76–100 years old) post mortem and found that of 61 participants meeting neuropathologic criteria for AD, those with brain infarcts had poorer cognitive function and higher prevalence of dementia than those without them. Perhaps most striking, lacunar infarcts in the basal ganglia, thalamus, or deep white matter were associated with an odds ratio for developing dementia of 20.7.

Zanetti and colleagues[58] studied 400 community-dwellers (≥65 years old) and found that of 65 individuals diagnosed with MCI (31 MCI-a, 34 MCI-md), 20 (31%)

progressed to dementia over 3 years of follow-up. Specifically, those diagnosed with MCI-md converted to VaD, whereas those diagnosed with MCI-a converted to AD. Similar findings, often from studies occurring outside the United States (eg, Italy, China, England), have led some researchers to conceptualize MCI-a as subsyndromal AD, and MCI-md as subsyndromal VaD. Others have argued that most cases of dementia result from a combination of both degenerative AD components and vascular factors: so-called mixed pathologies.[59]

The extent to which AD and VaD are truly independent remains unclear. An example of this complexity involves homocysteine, a byproduct of vitamins B_6 (pyridoxine), B_{12}, and folate metabolism, and a risk factor for vascular damage. When these substances are inadequate, homocysteine levels become increased, which in turn increases the risk for both vascular events and AD. A link between increased plasma homocysteine and poorer cognitive performance has been revealed repeatedly.[60–62]

Li and colleagues[55] replicated an earlier study[63] of the impact of treating VRF such as hypertension, diabetes, cerebrovascular disease, and hypercholesterolemia, on subsequent progression from MCI to AD over 5 years. Treatment was broadly operationalized to include behavioral factors such as smoking/alcohol cessation and diet modification. Of 837 individuals ($\geq$55 years old) diagnosed with MCI at baseline, 298 had progressed to AD (7.1% annually), whereas 352 (8.4% annually) remained stable. Those with VRF declined more rapidly and were at increased risk for AD conversion. Conversely, this risk was significantly reduced when VRF were being controlled with medication, behavioral change, or both.

Most recently, a group of 22 investigators joined forces to produce a comprehensive, 48-page scientific statement informed by review of 20 years of publications (1990–2010) documenting vascular contributions to MCI and dementia.[64] The investigators advocated for characterizing cognitive syndromes associated with vascular disease based on neuropsychological testing (to identify cognitive disorder) and neuroimaging (to identify lesions/infarcts). Vascular cognitive impairment (VCI) was the preferred umbrella term to classify all forms of cognitive disorder associated with cerebrovascular disease. It was defined as "a syndrome with evidence of clinical stroke or subclinical vascular brain injury and cognitive impairment affecting at least one cognitive domain...the most severe form of VCI is VaD."[(p2677)] Like MCI, VCI can affect multiple cognitive domains, including memory, although executive dysfunction has been considered a particularly salient feature. Analogous to the idea that MCI-a may be a mild subtype of AD, vascular mild cognitive impairment was also proposed as a potential precursor to VaD. This nomenclature continues to be refined and validated.

As future research attempts to elucidate their interrelationships more clearly, in practice, ongoing monitoring and management of cardiovascular factors is strongly indicated. Such factors are particularly amenable to behavioral interventions that encourage cost-effective, lifestyle-based patient self-management (eg, smoking cessation, diet modification, daily exercise). This self-management should be encouraged in patients and their families, with referral to interdisciplinary providers when possible (eg, clinical psychologists, nutritionists).

MANAGEMENT GOALS

Management goals and options depend largely on the presumptive cause of MCI. Reversible issues such as depression or overmedication can be addressed directly, as can improved control of chronic comorbidities and VRF. Caregivers and patients should be empowered to restructure activities and their environment in a manner that maximizes independence, including their ability to monitor illness from home.

This strategy can include fingersticks, blood pressure cuffs, and scales for weight management. Clinicians should strive to develop a collaborative, trusting alliance that allows for open, ongoing dialogue about sensitive topics such as establishing safety nets in case MCI progresses. Seven concrete goals of MCI management are listed in **Table 1**.

Although less straightforward, perhaps the ultimate MCI management goal is fostering acceptance, by both patients and families, that they may never experience their normal life prediagnosis again. Achieving this goal can require an extremely difficult, painful, and slow process, including high tolerance for ambiguity and a readjustment of expectations. Caregivers may need to repeat things more often than they would like. Patients may recognize they are not as competent as they once were. Family roles likely shift. Although frustration is inevitable, enhancing patient and family understanding of MCI and its variable nature can facilitate acceptance of its characteristic limitations. Provision of evidence-based resources and referral to community-based disease-specific advocacy groups may support this process and reduce anxiety. For patients and their families, adjusting expectations may prove the most challenging yet rewarding aspect of preserving their quality of life.

PHARMACOLOGIC STRATEGIES

There are no pharmacologic agents specifically approved to target MCI.[65] Rather, cholinesterase inhibitors (ChEIs) such as donepezil, rivastigmine, and galantamine, approved for treating symptomatic mild to moderate AD, have been examined in terms of efficacy for delaying or even preventing progression or conversion from MCI to AD. A 2007 study reviewed 8 randomized clinical trials (3 published, 5 unpublished); 3 of donepezil, 3 of galantamine, and 2 of rivastigmine. Trial duration ranged from 24 weeks to 3 years. The primary outcome measure was MCI conversion to

Table 1 Management goals	
Goal	**Examples**
Establish collaborative therapeutic alliance with patient and caregiver	Transparency when answering questions and admitting uncertainty. Willingness to negotiate based on patient preferences.
MCI reversal when possible	Reduce medications. Treat underlying conditions including mood.
Stabilize comorbid conditions	Address comorbidities, including vascular factors. Present options. Negotiate risk-benefit profiles. Clarify trade-offs.
Address both physical and mental health of patient and caregiver	Exercise, nutrition, sleep, meaningful engagement. (cognitive/social). Refer to community resources, including support groups/counseling.
Facilitate independence and quality of life	Empower to self-manage. Simplify environment. Reduce medication frequency/quantity. Use of technology.
Establish safety net in case of progression	Legal/financial considerations. Driving. Retirement. Advance directives.
Ongoing vigilance	Regular follow-up to reassess: cognition, function, mood, behavior, physical health, caregiver burden.

AD. No significant differences in the probability of such conversion between treatment and placebo groups were found.[66] Consistent with the clinical heterogeneity alluded to earlier, enrollment criteria were comparable in terms of instrument (ie, CDR, MMSE) but cutoff scores varied. In terms of outcomes, drug efficacy was determined with 38 different measures in cognitive, global/clinical, ADL, neuropsychiatric, and neuroimaging categories.

Most relevant from a management standpoint, in 3 of the 4 trials providing data on adverse events (AEs), fewer treatment group participants completed the studies than those assigned to placebo. Discontinuation rates were 21% to 24% among treatment recipients, and 7% to 13% among those receiving placebo. Therefore, the degree that investigators were truly blind is also questionable.

Of the 5 studies reporting death rates and group assignment, 27 deaths occurred among treatment group members (total n = 1842), whereas 19 were reported among placebo recipients (total n = 1880). In the only trial to report cause of death for both study arms, an unpublished galantamine trial, 6 deaths occurred in the treatment group, including 2 suicides, whereas 1 death occurred in the placebo condition (arrhythmia).

Of the 3 published randomized controlled trials (RCTs) reviewed, only 1 reported AE and discontinuation information. In each of the 3 unpublished studies reviewed, nearly 25% of treatment group participants discontinued their study participation because of AEs. This result seems noteworthy, given the potential for bias in industry-sponsored medication trials. Often, results indicating questionable therapeutic efficacy and frequent AEs are not published. The fact that unpublished studies are not peer reviewed lends further uncertainty regarding the rigor of measures used.

An unpublished trial of rivastigmine, from the review mentioned earlier, was subsequently published (InDDEx study).[67] Progression to AD was monitored over 4 years of follow-up for 1018 enrolled patients (508 rivastigmine, 504 placebo). Compared with individuals receiving placebo, slightly fewer treatment group participants progressed to AD (17.3% vs 21.4%), although there were no significant between-group differences on cognitive test performance from baseline to end point. Regarding safety, a higher incidence of more serious AEs (SAEs) was reported in the placebo condition (155 vs 141; 30.5% vs 27.9%). Cholinergic side effects (explained later) were most common and 2 to 4 times higher in the rivastigmine group. In a different study, donepezil plus vitamin E showed no benefit for delaying MCI-a conversion to AD over 3 years.[68]

Conversely, a 2009 meta-analysis of long-term use of ChEIs reported a 25% reduction in risk of progression from MCI to AD among a robust total sample size (3574 participants; 1784 treatment, 1790 placebo).[69] Although impressive in number, such findings should be interpreted with caution given the heterogeneity discussed thus far, perhaps most evident in the research study selection process. Initially, 173 studies were retrieved and only 10 were RCTs (6 published, 4 unpublished). Of these studies, only 3 met inclusion criteria (double-blind, placebo-controlled, RCTs of ChEIs, and primary outcome = delay of progression from predementia stages to AD), further evidence of the study design inconsistency that plagues the MCI literature.

Potential to delay disease progression in patients already diagnosed with AD has been evaluated with 2 other pharmacologic agents; memantine (N-methyl-D-aspartate receptor antagonist [NMDA]) and selegiline (monoamine oxidase inhibitor [MAOI]). An RCT found selegiline and α-tocopherol (vitamin E), both independently and in combination, to be efficacious for delaying disease progression among elders with moderately severe AD impairment.[70] Among trials of memantine, most of which have lasted 6 months, some but not all have shown small benefit among those with moderate to severe AD, with good tolerability.[71] Evaluation of appropriateness for MCI remains scant. In an evaluation across the dementia continuum, Winblad and Jelic[72] found that memantine was not effective for MCI or mild AD. A smaller study of 60 participants (50–79 years old) with age-associated memory impairment[73] revealed some benefit of memantine for attention and information processing speed but not memory.

What can be safely concluded from this discussion? It seems that ChEIs may be used interchangeably (ie, drug class effect) and may show modest symptomatic efficacy in MCI for up to 1 year. Evidence for any sustained impact beyond this time frame is limited. Given the mixed evidence on toxicity, patient tolerance should be closely monitored. Gastrointestinal cholinergic side effects, including nausea, vomiting, anorexia, weight loss, and diarrhea, have been the most common problems associated with ChEIs. Others include nightmares, cramping, and bradycardia. The efficacy of non-ChEI pharmacologic agents such as memantine, selegiline, and statins has not been compelling. Nor have studies of herbs and supplements such as gingko biloba, ginseng, folic acid, antioxidants, fish oil, and vitamin E.[74] Most of these trials included only patients with AD and not MCI. Nevertheless, off-label usage does occur in practice with older patients diagnosed with MCI.[65] Before prescribing these agents, clinicians should disclose to patients and caregivers that they are not approved for this use and briefly explain what this means in jargon-free language.

Medications to Avoid

The Beers Criteria for Potentially Inappropriate Medication use in Older Adults (ie, Beers list)[75] serves as an excellent clinical reference for minimizing adverse drug-drug interactions and related problems caused by polypharmacy. Such considerations are of paramount importance when managing older patients. Anticholinergic medications such as oxybutynin, commonly prescribed by urologists and primary care physicians to treat incontinence among the aged, are especially problematic and should not be used in combination with ChEIs. Significant anticholinergic side effects can include ataxia and tachycardia and can also affect the central nervous system. The latter may prompt a host of untoward consequences that mimic cognitive symptoms typical of delirium (eg, confusion, disorientation, agitation) or even dementia (eg, memory and concentration difficulty, brain fog, incoherent speech, visual/auditory/sensory hallucinations). Statins, β-blockers, certain eye drops, and even over-the-counter (OTC) sleep agents have also been associated with cognitive impairment. Careful adjustment, including discontinuation, of problematic medications can lead to remarkable improvement in cognition.

Simplifying Medication Regimens

In addition to safety, it is important to consider discontinuing medications of questionable long-term benefit, particularly for elderly patients. Statins are a classic example. Although they were initially touted for possible neuroprotective benefits and therefore potentially indicated for treatment of AD/MCI, a recent meta-analysis of RCTs showed that their efficacy has not been proved.[76] Non-RCT evidence remains mixed both for possible benefits and adverse effect on cognition and quality of life.[77–81] By negotiating effectively with patients and families, clinicians can better understand how to maximize their adherence and prioritize their treatment goals. Regarding the oxybutynin example, clinicians might ask patients presenting with bladder leakage and memory complaints which is more important: to be dry or to remember? The decision of which medication to discontinue can thus be guided by patient preference.

Timing, Dosage, and Frequency

As a rule, it is advisable to minimize the number and frequency of medications used. In practice, ideal medication dosing may be compromised if adherence becomes difficult. Once-a-day dosage regimens can improve the likelihood of consistent adherence. Timing of administration should coalesce with patients' everyday routines to the extent possible; sedating agents should be taken before bedtime, those that must be taken after meals should be administered after breakfast or lunch. Given the challenges of managing drug-drug interactions and polypharmacy among geriatric patients, sleep hygiene is preferred over sleep agents, especially those sold OTC (ie, Tylenol PM, Benadryl), which tend to have anticholinergic side effects. Sleep deprivation can affect cognition and must be managed.

NONPHARMACOLOGIC STRATEGIES
Behavioral Interventions

In light of the limited pharmacotherapeutic efficacy alluded to earlier, behavioral interventions have also been tested. Emerging evidence suggests that modifiable psychological factors such as mood and beliefs, both amenable to counseling approaches, may play a role in level and rapidity of cognitive decline.[82] Purpose in life, measured by a validated 10-item scale (eg, I have a sense of direction and purpose in life; I am an active person in carrying out the plans I set for myself), has shown an independent, protective impact on cognition, even in research models including other potential contributors such as number of chronic physical illnesses (eg, stroke, diabetes mellitus, hypertension).[83] Level of sociability and social network size, likely related to level of isolation, have also been linked to positive cognitive outcomes.[84,85] Research attempts to elucidate the physiologic effect of these and related psychological factors have shown promise and have included posited biomarkers for cognitive decline such as immunologic and vascular factors.[86,87] Although articulated (and measured) in multiple ways, existential concerns are increasingly prevalent among geriatric patients as they live out their final years. Social support can provide relief and buffer cognitive impact.

Cognitive Interventions

Enduring, observable, treatment effects have been reported for cognitive interventions with healthy elders.[88] Three particular types (cognitive stimulation [CS], cognitive training [CT] and cognitive rehabilitation [CR]) are the most common and well researched. CS aims to improve cognitive and social function rather broadly. CT is task-specific (eg, memory, attention, ADL, problem solving) and aims to maintain or even improve abilities in the hope that they may transfer to similar but untrained real-life tasks. CR is similar to CT but places stronger emphasis on everyday contexts and functioning. In a recent review, Kurz and colleagues[89] meta-analyzed 33 studies: 20 CS and 13 CT/CR. CS intervention was most common in long-term care settings and implemented with patients diagnosed with dementia. CT/CR treatment was usually provided to persons diagnosed with MCI and occurred in memory clinics or research centers.

Overall, there was some evidence for improvement with MCI. Treatment effects were short-lived (ie, <6 months), although 1 study reported gains maintained at 2-year follow-up.[90] Most relevant to patient management, it remains unclear to what extent laboratory-based improvement translates to everyday tasks.[91] The latter are often not included in research designs. Evidence of success has often been measured with cognitive symptoms. Although such data are meaningful and conducive to empirical measurement, in terms of clinical management, some have suggested that conversion to dementia or symptom progression may be more useful outcome measures.[92]

Although such designs target cognition, positive impact on mood may occur even without cognitive improvement. In some cases, participants' perceived memory capability increased after training, although this was not corroborated by objective memory testing.[93] Are these secondary outcome benefits clinically meaningful or significant? This question should be addressed on an individual case basis, and clinicians should facilitate such discussion with patients and families when possible.

A similar conclusion was reported by investigators in a comprehensive, Cochrane review of nearly 40 years of published literature (1970–2007) assessing the effectiveness of CT with both cognitively healthy and cognitively impaired older adults.[46] Only 3 of 36 RCTs included individuals diagnosed with MCI. Methodological heterogeneity also limited data pooling significantly. Limitations aside, the investigators did conclude that there was evidence that cognitive interventions targeting memory do show significant training gains. Whether or not this impact was intervention-specific remains less clear, because improvement was no greater than that among active control (ie, alternative treatment) participants. How can this finding be explained? It seems that mental engagement, itself, may exert a role on both mood and performance. Although beyond the scope of this article, evidence for a link between mood, perceived competence, and performance has been shown repeatedly across self-efficacy research in cognitive and other behavioral domains, including memory.[94]

Although duration of improvement and generalizability to everyday functional tasks are debatable, some studies of cognitive interventions have reported depressive symptom reduction rates as high as 50%, thus rivaling psychotropic treatment efficacy.[89] Because of methodological challenges (eg, no control group or nonspecific support group conditions) and heterogeneity, it remains unclear to what extent mood boosts are caused by positive engagement with peers and other caring, interested parties, all of whom are focused on facilitating improvement. Although challenging to measure, this therapeutic milieu has been described extensively by psychiatrists and psychologists when referring to nonspecific treatment factors present in counseling group dynamics.[95] Regardless, the mood-enhancing qualities of such training suggest that it could be provided more routinely, including as adjunct to pharmacologic treatment, with minimal risk of untoward consequences. The fact that it is not likely related to skepticism and economic constraints more than evidence.

Useful Field of View and Cognitive Processing Speed

Useful field of view (UFOV) testing and cognitive processing speed represent a slightly different area of CT that has primarily targeted driving-related skills. Data have been mixed, although UFOV has been considered a valid and reliable index for predicting driving performance and safety, and therefore a good screening tool for potentially unsafe drivers.[96] Cognitive processing speed, as measured by UFOV, has been shown to predict driving cessation, even when controlling for vision, health, and physical performance.[97–99]

A recent 3-year study[100] examined the efficacy of cognitive processing speed training for elders with poor UFOV scores, and thus at higher risk for at-fault crashes and subsequent decline in mobility. After training, their scores on cognitive outcome measures were indistinguishable from those of a control group with good baseline UFOV scores. Another study[88] reported maintenance of UFOV improvements for 5 years after training.

Based on the preponderance of evidence, it seems that the success of cognitive interventions depends on the degree to which they are individually tailored. Because functional impairment, by definition, is generally limited in MCI, CR or CT programs seem more appropriate than CS. However, a growing body of evidence shows that patients with MCI may lose skills necessary for more complex instrumental ADL (IADL) such as financial management, medication adherence, and safe driving; suggesting that such abilities may be less preserved than once believed.[101,102]

Peres and colleagues[17] attempted to quantify the impact of restricted IADL (telephone, transportation, medication, financial management) on MCI reversal and conversion to AD in a sample of 1517 participants (≥65 years old) at 8-year and 10-year follow-up. Of the 285 participants diagnosed with MCI at baseline, 15.2% developed dementia within 2 years. Over this same time frame, those who were IADL-restricted were nearly 4 times more likely to convert to dementia than those who were not (30.7% vs 7.8%). Furthermore, the investigators reported IADL restriction reduced the likelihood of reverting to normal cognitive status. Reversal was more than 3 times as likely for those whose IADL were not restricted (34.7% vs 10.7%).

A population-based study of 1737 community-dwellers (≥65 years old) focused on 7 IADL; traveling, shopping, meal preparation, housework, medication, financial management, and using the telephone.[103] Those diagnosed with MCI were more likely to show impairment in at least 1 IADL compared with controls without an MCI diagnosis. Better memory and executive functioning were associated with lower odds of IADL impairment. Those diagnosed with amnestic MCI-md were most likely to show impairment in all IADL.

Another study went a step further in terms of specificity. Financial management decrements were associated with diagnosis of MCI-a, whereas limited ability in activities related to health and safety (eg, awareness of own health status, ability to assess health problems, dealing with medical emergencies, and knowledge of healthy behaviors) were linked to MCI-na.[104] These data suggest that IADL may provide useful clinical information about cognitive status. Ongoing monitoring is therefore indicated.

Counseling/Psychotherapy

A high prevalence of geriatric depression and anxiety makes referral for evidence-based psychotherapy potentially appropriate.[105] In the case of degenerative disease, in which family roles must often be adjusted, it is not uncommon for diagnosis to be followed by the resurfacing of conflict and discord that have otherwise remained unaddressed by families for years. This situation can impede clinical management and even be dangerous. Clinical geropsychologists have specific training and expertise to manage such difficulties via individual, couples, or group counseling. Sessions are often conducted on a weekly basis. Less-intensive, monthly or biweekly community-based support groups may also be available. The emergence of interdisciplinary, team-based approaches and integrated health care delivery systems bodes well for optimal biopsychosocial treatment. Nonetheless, bias, stigma, and other barriers remain. When presenting counseling options to patients and families, discussion should include possible insurance-related reimbursement and time (session duration) limitations. Challenges notwithstanding, clinicians ideally have trusted behavioral health colleagues to whom they can comfortably refer and with whom they can coordinate regularly to ensure ongoing, efficient clinical monitoring.

SELF-MANAGEMENT STRATEGIES

What can patients and their caregivers do to independently manage their own health? As mentioned earlier, adequately informed and educated patients and families can self-monitor for subtle factors that may affect cognition with advancing age. Dehydration is a common example. Aging patients may lose thirst drive or intentionally limit fluid intake to avoid continence problems. This situation can lead to confusion and subsequent emergency room visits, which may have been preventable. Inadequate rest or sleep deprivation may also compromise cognition. Complicating matters, OTC sleep medications often have anticholinergic effects, which can impair attention and memory. Establishing trust with patients can facilitate ongoing dialogue and monitoring both within and outside the clinic setting. In the next sections, the efficacy of more specific self-management strategies is examined.

Lifestyle

Implicit in research on cognitive plasticity has been the idea that lifestyle, including engagement in mentally and physically challenging activities (eg, leisure, professional), can contribute to cognitive vitality in later life. Exemplifying this notion is the popular adage, "use it or lose it." Kramer and colleagues[106] tested this idea by reviewing the related literature. Vastly diverse study designs precluded any firm conclusions, but the adage did receive some empirical support. Intellectually challenging and complex environments and engagement in novel tasks may enhance cognition. This association was clearer when measured by general (ie, MMSE) rather than specific measures of cognitive decline and was strongest when measured over the span of several decades. Physical fitness, described in more detail in the next section, also conferred a positive impact on cognition, particularly when the duration of exercise was at least 30 minutes.

Physical Fitness

Evidence for the benefit of physical activity on cognitive aging dates back nearly half a century.[107] A meta-analysis of longitudinal studies conducted between 1966 and 2001 showed cognitive benefits from aerobic fitness among cognitively intact elders.[108] This finding was most apparent for tasks requiring executive control, including driving.[109] Maximal benefit was conferred by fitness programs combining strength, flexibility, and cardiovascular training. Some have deduced from these findings that physical exercise may serve a prophylactic purpose in healthy elders.[106] Similar to the CT literature reviewed earlier, evidence of benefit for individuals already diagnosed with MCI is limited.

Nutrition

Diet has been targeted for MCI self-management. Consumption of fish, particularly fatty varieties such as salmon or mackerel, has been touted as an excellent source of health-promoting long-chain omega-3 fatty acids. Theoretically, they may improve cerebral blood flow, mitigate inflammation, and reduce amyloid aggregation, all posited biomarkers for dementia. Some empirical evidence has supported the idea that weekly fish consumption may protect against age-associated cognitive decline.[110] In a systematic review of all related articles published over nearly 3 decades (1980–2008), Fotuhi and colleagues[111] analyzed 11 observational studies and 4 clinical trials. Evidence was mixed. Those measuring cognitive impairment as the outcome were found to show a modest benefit of fish consumption or omega-3 fatty acid supplements, albeit short-lived, whereas those studies examining possible prevention or treatment of dementia did not show benefit. More broadly, the so-called Mediterranean diet, varied and rich in fruits and vegetables, whole grains, lean proteins, olive oil, and moderate wine consumption, and low in saturated fats, has been endorsed by popular culture and supported by some research.[112]

Alcohol

Although not without controversy, alcohol consumption has been studied extensively. Purported cardiovascular benefit from alcohol consumption has spawned analogue attempts to decipher a similar impact on cognition. Ability to draw firm conclusions based on literature reviews and meta-analyses is challenged by inconsistent methodologies. Examination of various alcohol consumption patterns (often tied to cultural practices, including diet) has yielded mixed results. Although benefits of wine seem to be better established than those of either beer or liquor, studies often do not distinguish among grape type or even wine color (ie, red/white/rosé). Furthermore, comparisons of wine consumers and abstainers often do not specify whether abstinence refers to a lifelong behavioral pattern or a shift at some point in life, perhaps as a response to negative outcomes related to previous misuse, and any subsequent damage caused by such use.

In a recent review of 19 studies examining the relationship between alcohol and AD,[113] 7 showed that consumption decreased AD risk, 3 showed it increased risk, and 9 showed no significant relationship. Fewer data exist on alcohol and MCI although some evidence suggests that moderate alcohol consumption (ie, 1 drink or 15 g of alcohol/d), particularly wine, may delay rate of progression to AD.[114]

Technology

Depending on level of impairment, automated bill payments and notifications may extend patients' ability to remain independent. Computer programs (ie, Skype), cellular phones, mobile applications, and related electronic devices may help manage weekly schedules and provide reminders of appointments, names, and other information, and enable monitoring of patients, if necessary, when they are left alone or unsupervised. Such mechanisms may reduce daily pressures and enhance quality of life for both patients and caregivers. Self-driving cars are being tested in several US cities, although their widespread availability in the near future is unlikely.

Self-Management Summary

In light of the evidence for self-management strategies reviewed thus far, reasonable recommendations include a balanced and varied diet that emphasizes fish, fruits, and vegetables; weekly (if not daily) physical exercise of 20-to-30 minute duration; good sleep hygiene; adequate hydration; and engagement in pleasurable cognitive (ie, reading, writing, Internet use) and social activity. For those already consuming moderate alcohol, this can be continued (ie, 1 drink/d). The evidence does not support recommending abstainers to begin drinking, but does suggest heavier consumers of alcohol should reduce their intake. Because evidence of benefit for most of these approaches has been mixed, quality-of-life implications of these and other lifestyle choices should be evaluated based on individual patient preferences. Technology may be used as a compensatory strategy for memory lapses or other cognitive problems that pose challenges to everyday functioning, and can facilitate communication between patients and family members.

EVALUATION, ADJUSTMENT, RECURRENCE
Frequency of Follow-Up

The nature of MCI suggests that symptom severity likely fluctuates. Determining appropriate intervals between clinical visits can therefore be highly variable. Many clinicians leave the decision up to the patient/family to return if and when they notice decline. Generally, follow-up appointments are advised at 6 to 12 months. In cases in which MCI is not reversible and does represent the early stage of neurodegeneration, impending decline is likely insidious and unlikely detectable before 6 months or a year. In cases in which reliable caregivers are absent, more frequent follow-up such as every 3 months is prudent. The main premise is to empower patients and caregivers to actively monitor any progression or decline between visits. IADL performance is a standard metric that they can use.

DISCUSSION

We hope that it is clear from this review that although the last decade has seen solid progress, there remains much to uncover about all aspects of MCI: cause, diagnosis, management, and treatment. Just as Petersen and colleagues[6] described more than a decade ago, operationalization challenges, lack of consensus, and surplus of conflicting empirical evidence necessitate sensitive clinical judgment. As frustrating as the unknown may seem to clinicians, it is all the more unsettling for the patients whom they must manage. We conclude, therefore, with several ethical considerations to guide and optimize a shared treatment and decision-making process.

Diagnostic Disclosure

When should diagnosis occur? How and to whom should diagnosis be disclosed? The uncertainties linked to MCI and its future course, and diversity of patient preferences, make specific, one-size-fits-all recommendations for diagnostic disclosure inappropriate. Based on the level of evidence, there are no easy answers. Theoretically, earlier assessment and documentation of MCI can be important if it leads to accurate detection, ongoing monitoring, and if appropriate, earlier treatment. Such a proactive stance may aid clinicians in delaying progression to a more serious cognitive condition (ie, AD) and elicit conversation, both with and among patients and family members, about reducing work obligations and retirement planning. This discussion can include sensitive, difficult-to-face topics such as new approaches to financial management if and when they become necessary. Open disclosure allows for maximum input from patients in terms of advance directives and goals of care. Given its sensitive nature, diagnosis should be delivered in person, not by telephone or mail.

Although this rationale may seem prudent, there are legal and ethical issues to consider, such as stigma and insurability, especially given the limits of treatment options. Furthermore, MCI, even if accurately diagnosed, may not signify a progressive, degenerative process. As shown earlier, with time, symptoms may remit and cognition may return to premorbid normal levels. Given this possibility, planning for retirement or changes in occupational status may be premature and unwarranted. Such concerns may trigger unnecessary anxiety and other psychological harm.

In the absence of a gold standard, pros and cons of disclosure should be considered on a case-by-case basis. Openness and clarity are beneficial to both patients and caregivers, with some evidence that anxiety and depressive symptoms remain stable or even decline after diagnosis.[115] This finding is largely consistent with anecdotal evidence from the authors' clinical experience. Patients and their caregivers consistently express preference and appreciation for transparency, even if this means that clinicians must admit to uncertainty and limited scientific knowledge and treatment options.

Clinicians should be prepared for questions about genetic testing and research participation. We recommend against testing unless there is a strong family history of early-onset dementia (ie, parent diagnosed before 65 years old) corresponding to a patient's MCI diagnosed 10 years earlier. Encouraging research participation is reasonable. However, to avoid risks of delay in appropriate treatment, patients should continue to be monitored independently of a particular study.

Depression and Anxiety

Epidemiologic studies have reported unclear roles for depression and other psychiatric symptoms in predicting MCI conversion to dementia. Successful management approaches likely differ, case by case, depending on the relationship (ie, cause or effect) between such signs and symptoms and MCI. For example, is depression contributing to MCI and therefore a potentially reversible antecedent? Or, is it a response to awareness of the cognitively impaired state? Regardless of direction, mood concerns should be monitored and treated, especially among older patients. Cognitive aging research on healthy community-dwellers has documented the influence of affective states on perceived memory competence and subsequent performance.[116–118] Although depression can interfere with both cognitive and functional ability, its relationship to MCI is difficult to ascertain because exclusion of individuals with these and other common psychiatric symptoms (eg, anxiety) is frequent within MCI-related literature.[55,119–121] Given that estimates of forgetting frequency and other self-report memory assessments are often intertwined with depression, effectively managing mood (ie, depression/anxiety) with or without medications may have a beneficial effect on cognition. Depressive symptoms and cognitive dysfunction, both individually and in combination, can predict all-cause mortality,[122] and suicide completion is one such cause for which older adults are at greatest risk across the globe.[123]

Suicide

Suicide completion increases with age,[124] and older white men are the most successful, often using firearms.[125] Concerned clinicians face several challenges. First, open enquiry into risks and hazards of gun ownership, both via research and clinical practice, is facing increased political interference.[126] In addition, older patients are less likely to endorse affective symptoms (eg, depression) and more likely to show cognitive changes, somatic symptoms, and loss of interest.[127] Rates of depression among older adults who have killed themselves have been as high as 85%.[128] Specific contributing factors include hopelessness,[129] change in medical status, and perceived burden to others[130]; all common correlates of neurodegenerative processes such as cognitive impairment and dementia. The most compelling support for monitoring mood may be that among older people who commit suicide, the percentage who have seen their primary care physician within a month before their death has been estimated at 70%.[131] There are multiple interpretive explanations for this rate but the need for clinicians to remain vigilant is unequivocal.

At minimum, clinicians should assess for suicidal ideation when screening for emotionally depression. Patients are often relieved when the topic is broached, and concern that doing so may plant or encourage the idea is unwarranted. Clinical judgment should inform whether patients are assessed alongside caregivers or separately, although the latter is often advised when discussing emotionally delicate material.[132] Brief, validated instruments are easy to administer and can help guide assessment.[133]

Legal and Financial Matters

Enquiry into patients' and their families' level of preparedness in terms of possible functional decline, even if it may not occur for some time, or at all, is advisable. This strategy may elicit conversation and even concrete steps toward preparation of legal documents such as living wills, establishing a durable power of attorney, a medical proxy, and any other advance directives. Again, although diagnosis does not guarantee any change in impairment level, these are important topics to address nonetheless. Such discussion may morph into hypothetical worst-case scenarios and their implications, such as creating a safety net for managing finances and medications if patients are no longer able to do so independently. This discussion can culminate with a focus on how to determine when patients should reconsider their profession, independent driving, and living arrangements (eg, at home in community vs institutionalization), and as a corollary to this, who will be responsible for making such determinations. Generally, patients and caregivers show preferences for discussion and recommendations to occur early on, ideally at diagnosis.[22]

Complex IADL Function

Basic ADL such as dressing or bathing are comparable across cultures and generally intact among those with MCI. However, more complex IADL may not be intact, and function should therefore be monitored frequently.[134] IADL are often influenced by culture-specific norms that apply to variables such as education, socioeconomic status, and gender. Clinical implications can be subtle yet powerful, as shown by the following example. In some cultures, gender norms may result in men who never cook or assume responsibility for maintaining household order, or women who never drive or manage finances. In such cases, spouses or family members of the opposite sex face an especially challenging role adjustment as they strive to compensate for patients whose MCI symptoms (and subsequent dependence) progress.

Perhaps the ultimate IADL is driving. Some have argued that cognitive performance is the strongest predictor of subsequent driving limitations.[135] Research in this area has mainly explored potential links between AD and risk of automobile crash, yielding mixed results.[136–139] Evidence of a link between diminished driving capacity and MCI is limited. In part, this situation may be caused by the methodological challenge of measuring this relationship in a linear fashion. In practice, as impaired patients deteriorate, family often intervenes by limiting but not necessarily prohibiting their driving. The resulting decreased driving exposure (ie, frequency and distance) often reduces crash rates but makes accurate tests of the impairment-driving relationship difficult.

Among the few studies exploring the driving-MCI link, one[140] compared crash rates of 63 drivers with a CDR score of very mild or mild impairment with a control group and found no significant difference over the previous 5 years. Wadley and colleagues[141] found that those with MCI showed more subtle challenges in driving, and their performance of discrete driving behaviors (eg, left turn) was more often objectively rated less than optimal compared with a control group of neurocognitively normal drivers. Although a statistically significant difference, members of the control group also received less than optimal ratings on driving behaviors. Clinical significance of this result is therefore debatable.

SUMMARY

MCI is perhaps best characterized by uncertainty (**Table 2**). This situation constitutes a major challenge to patients, their families, and clinicians alike. It is our experience that many principles of behavioral science are therefore particularly helpful in MCI management. Empathic, clear communication about what patients and families may expect, available options, and limitations, is crucial. Education about self-monitoring between clinic visits can build trust and a sense of empowerment. Such efforts may maximize the likelihood of open dialogue and accurate reporting of symptom (and disease) progression at subsequent follow-up appointments. Clinical acumen is especially vital to older patients for whom cognitive impairment is suspected and the temptation to view intervention as futile is increased, even within the medical community. In the face of prognostic and diagnostic uncertainty, it is

Table 2
Management strategies

Intervention	Unknown or No Evidence for Benefit in MCI	Some Evidence	Strong Evidence
Pharmacologic			
ChEIs (donepezil, rivastigmine, galantamine, tacrine[a])		X	No
NMDA receptor blocker (memantine)	X		No
MAOI (selegiline)	X		No
Statins		X	No
Herbals and supplements			
Vitamin E (α-tocopherol)	X		No
Gingko biloba	X		No
Ginseng	X		No
B_{12}	X		No
B_6-Pyridoxine	X		No
Folate	X		No
B_1-Thiamine	X		No
Omega-3 fatty acids		X	No
Reduce vascular risk		X	No
Lifestyle (ie, nutrition, Mediterranean diet, exercise, alcohol, sleep)		X	No
CT (ie, CR, CS, UFOV)		X	No
Psychotherapy/counseling	X		No

[a] Discontinued because of toxicity.

precisely this sensitivity that should inform patient-centered, shared clinical decision making. Evidence linking skillful communication to positive clinical outcomes, including patient satisfaction and adherence to medical regimens, has been shown by a robust empirical literature spanning more than half a century.[142–144] Despite their well-documented relevance, medical training in these interpersonal aspects of care remains limited.

As a result, clinicians may unknowingly discourage patients and their families from active participation in their own care. Although often inadvertent, this situation can have significant management implications. Because much is unknown about the course and timing of degenerative disease, the need for clinicians to collaboratively involve families and patients cannot be overemphasized. In some cases, families may seek out alternative therapies (eg, coconut water) on their own. If no harm is occurring, scientific evidence for what patients and families may believe is helpful may not be overly important. However, dismissing their ideas can be damaging. Clinicians should acknowledge such efforts, have frank conversation about level of evidence and potential for financial exploitation, and show a willingness to remain open to follow-up discussion. Whichever clinical path MCI takes, attention to these dynamics can foster an efficient and enduring therapeutic alliance. In the face of prognostic uncertainty, MCI management effectiveness may be determined less by what clinicians do, and more by how they do it.

REFERENCES

1. Rubin EH, Morris JC, Grant EA, et al. Very mild senile dementia of the Alzheimer type: clinical assessment. Arch Neurol 1989;46(4):379–82.
2. Morris JC, McKeel DW Jr, Storandt M, et al. Very mild Alzheimer's disease: informant-based clinical, psychometric, and pathologic distinction from normal aging. Neurology 1991;41(4):469–78.
3. Flicker C, Ferris SH, Reisberg B. Mild cognitive impairment in the elderly: predictors of dementia. Neurology 1991;41(7):1006.
4. Petersen RC, Smith GE, Ivnik RJ, et al. Memory function in very early Alzheimer's. Neurology 1994;44(5):867.
5. Smith GE, Petersen RC, Parisi JE, et al. Definition, course, and outcome of mild cognitive impairment. Aging Neuropsychol Cognit 1996;3:131–47.
6. Petersen RC, Smith GE, Waring SC, et al. Mild cognitive impairment: clinical characterization and outcome. Arch Neurol 1999;56(3):303–8.
7. Morris JC, Storandt M, Miller JP, et al. Mild cognitive impairment represents early-stage Alzheimer disease. Arch Neurol 2001;58:397–405.
8. Solfrizzi V, Panza F, Colacicco AM, et al. Vascular risk factors, incidence of MCI, and rates of progression to dementia. Neurology 2004;63:1882–991.
9. Larrieu S, Letenneuer L, Orgogozo JM, et al. Incidence and outcome of mild cognitive impairment in a population-based cohort. Neurology 2002;59:1594–9.
10. Roberts R, Geda Y, Knopman D, et al. Men are more likely to have mild cognitive impairment than women: the Mayo Clinic study of aging. Paper presented at the American Academy of Neurology. Chicago, April 12–19, 2008.
11. Perri R, Serra L, Carelsimo GA, et al. Preclinical dementia: an Italian multicenter study on amnestic mild cognitive impairment. Dement Geriatr Cogn Disord 2007;23:289–300.
12. Manly JJ, Tang MX, Schupf N, et al. Frequency and course of mild cognitive impairment in a multiethnic community. Ann Neurol 2008;63(4):494–506.
13. Petersen RC, Stevens JC, Ganguli M, et al. Practice parameter: early detection of dementia: mild cognitive impairment (an evidence-based review). Report of the Quality Standards Subcommittee of the American Academy of Neurology. Neurology 2001;56:1133–42.
14. Saxton J, Snitz BE, Lopez OL, et al. Functional and cognitive criteria produce different rates of mild cognitive impairment and conversion to dementia. J Neurol Neurosurg Psychiatry 2009;80:737–43.
15. Ganguli M, Dodge HH, Shen C, et al. Mild cognitive impairment, amnestic type: an epidemiologic study. Neurology 2004;63:115–21.
16. Perri R, Carlesimo GA, Serra L, et al. When the amnestic mild cognitive impairment disappears. Cogn Behav Neurol 2009;22(2):109–16.
17. Peres K, Chrysostome V, Fabrigoule C, et al. Restriction in complex activities of daily living in MCI: impact on outcome. Neurology 2006;67:461–6.
18. Abner EL, Kryscio RJ, Cooper GE, et al. Mild cognitive impairment: statistical models of transition using longitudinal clinical data. Int J Alzheimers Dis 2012;2012:291920.
19. Winblad B, Palmer K, Kivipelto M, et al. Mild cognitive impairment-beyond controversies, towards a consensus: report of the International Working Group on Mild Cognitive Impairment. J Intern Med 2004;256:240–6.
20. Pearman A, Storandt M. Predictors of subjective memory in older adults. J Gerontol B Psychol Sci Soc Sci 2004;59:P4–6.

21. Lenehan ME, Klekociuk SZ, Summers MJ. Absence of a relationship between subjective memory complaint and objective memory impairment (MCI): is it time to abandon subjective memory complaint as an MCI diagnostic criterion? Int Psychogeriatr 2012;24(9):1505–14.

22. Widera E, Steenpass V, Marson D, et al. Finances in the older patient with cognitive impairment: he didn't want me to take over. JAMA 2011;305(7): 698–706.

23. Essig M, Buchem MA. Degenerative brain disease and aging. In: Hodler J, von Schulthess GK, Zollikofer CH, editors. Diseases of the brain, head & neck, spine 2012-2015. Milan (Italy): Springer; 2012. p. 58–66.

24. Folstein MF, Folstein SE, McHugh PR. Mini-mental state: a practical method for grading the cognitive state of patients for the clinician. J Psychiatr Res 1975; 12(3):189–98.

25. Ward A, Arrighi HM, Michels S, et al. Mild cognitive impairment: disparity of incidence and prevalence estimates. Alzheimers Dement 2012;8:14–21.

26. Albert MS, DeKosky ST, Dickson D, et al. The diagnosis of mild cognitive impairment due to Alzheimer's disease: recommendations from the National Institute on Ageing-Alzheimer's Association Workgroups on diagnostic guidelines for Alzheimer's disease. Alzheimers Dement 2011;7:270–9.

27. Petersen RC, Doody R, Kurz A, et al. Current concepts in mild cognitive impairment. Arch Neurol 2001;58(12):1985–92.

28. Schneider JA, Arvanitakis Z, Leurgans SE, et al. The neuropathology of probable Alzheimer disease and mild cognitive impairment. Ann Neurol 2009;66:200–8.

29. Galluzzi S, Cimaschi L, Ferrucci L, et al. Mild cognitive impairment: clinical features and review of screening instruments. Aging 2001;13(3):183–202.

30. Small GW, Kepe V, Ercoli LM, et al. PET of brain amyloid and tau in mild cognitive impairment. N Engl J Med 2006;355:2652–7.

31. Aizenstein HJ, Nebes R, Saxton JA, et al. Frequent amyloid deposition without significant cognitive impairment among the elderly. Arch Neurol 2008;65: 1509–17.

32. Frisoni GB, Prestia A, Zanetti O, et al. Markers of Alzheimer's disease in a population attending a memory clinic. Alzheimers Dement 2009;5(4):307–17.

33. Elias-Sonnenschein LS, Viechtbauer W, Ramakers IH, et al. Predictive value of APOE-4 allele for progression from MCI to AD-type dementia: a meta-analysis. J Neurol Neurosurg Psychiatry 2011;82:1149–56.

34. Guo LH, Alexopoulos P, Eisele T, et al. The National Institute on Aging-Alzheimer's Association research criteria for mild cognitive impairment due to Alzheimer's disease: predicting the outcome. Eur Arch Psychiatry Clin Neurosci 2013;263(4):325–33.

35. Devanand DP, Folz M, Gorlyn M, et al. Questionable dementia: clinical course and predictors of outcome. J Am Geriatr Soc 1997;45:321–8.

36. De Jager C, Blackwell AD, Budge MM, et al. Predicting cognitive decline in healthy older adults. Am J Geriatr Psychiatry 2005;13:735–40.

37. Daly E, Zaitchik D, Copeland M, et al. Predicting conversion to Alzheimer's using standardized clinical information. Arch Neurol 2000;57:675–80.

38. Hanninen T, Hallikainen M, Koivisto K, et al. A follow-up study of age-associated memory impairment: neuropsychological predictors of dementia. J Am Geriatr Soc 1995;43:1007–15.

39. Palmer K, Wang HY, Backman L, et al. Differential evolution of cognitive impairment in nondemented older persons: results from the Kungsholmen project. Am J Psychiatry 2002;159(3):436–42.

40. Wahlund LO, Pihlstrand E, Jonhagen ME. Mild cognitive impairment: experience from a memory clinic. Acta Neurol Scand Suppl 2003;179:21–4.
41. Wolf H, Grunwald M, Ecke GM, et al. The prognosis of mild cognitive impairment in the elderly. J Neural Transm 1998;54(Suppl):31–50.
42. Visser PJ, Verhey FR, Ponds RW, et al. Course of objective memory impairment in non-demented subjects attending a memory clinic and predictors of outcome. Int J Geriatr Psychiatry 2000;15:363–72.
43. Gauthier S, Touchon J. Mild cognitive impairment is not a clinical entity and should not be treated. Arch Neurol 2006;62:1164–6.
44. Graham JE, Rockwood K, Beattie BL, et al. Prevalence and severity of cognitive impairment with and without dementia in an elderly population. Lancet 1997; 349:1793–6.
45. Di Carlo A, Baldereschi M, Amaducci L, et al. Cognitive impairment without dementia in older people: prevalence, vascular risk factors, impact on disability: the Italian longitudinal study on aging. J Am Geriatr Soc 2000;48:775–82.
46. Martin M, Clare L, Altgassen AM, et al. Cognition-based interventions for healthy older people and people with mild cognitive impairment. Cochrane Database Syst Rev 2011;(1):CD006220. http://dx.doi.org/10.1002/14651858.CD006220.pub2.
47. Burke WJ, Miller JP, Rubin EH, et al. Reliability of the Washington University Clinical Dementia Rating Scale. Arch Neurol 1988;45(1):31–2.
48. Morris JC. The clinical dementia rating (CDR): current version and scoring rules. Neurology 1993;43(11):2412–4.
49. Reisberg B, Ferris SH, deLeon MJ, et al. The global deterioration scale for assessment of primary degenerative dementia. Am J Psychiatry 1982;139(9): 1136–9.
50. Schneider JA, Wilson RS, Bienias JL, et al. Cerebral infarctions and the likelihood of dementia from Alzheimer disease pathology. Neurology 2004;62:1148–55.
51. Binswanger O. Die Abgrenzung der allgemeinen progressiven Paralyse. Berl Kli Wochenschr 1894;31:1180–6 [in German].
52. Wiederkehr S, Simard M, Fortin C, et al. Comparability of the clinical diagnostic criteria for vascular dementia: a critical review part 1. J Neuropsychiatry Clin Neurosci 2008;20(2):150–61.
53. Panza F, D'Introno A, Colacicco AM, et al. Cognitive frailty: predementia syndrome and vascular risk factors. Neurobiol Aging 2006;27(7):933–40.
54. DiCarlo A, Lamassa M, Baldereschi M, et al. CIND and MCI in the Italian elderly: frequency, vascular risk factors, progression to dementia. Neurology 2007;68: 1909–16.
55. Li J, Wang YJ, Zhang M, et al. Vascular risk factors promote conversion from mild cognitive impairment to Alzheimer disease. Neurology 2011;76(17):1485–91.
56. Snowdon DA. Healthy aging and dementia: findings from the nun study. Ann Intern Med 2003;139:450–4.
57. Snowdon DA, Grainer LH, Mortimer JA, et al. Brain infarction and the clinical expression of Alzheimer disease: the Nun Study. JAMA 1997;277:813–7.
58. Zanetti M, Ballabio C, Abbate C, et al. Mild cognitive impairment subtypes and vascular dementia in community-dwelling elderly people: a 3-year follow-up study. J Am Geriatr Soc 2006;54:580–6.
59. Schneider JA, Arvanitakis Z, Bang W, et al. Mixed brain pathologies account for most dementia cases in community-dwelling older persons. Neurology 2007;69: 2197–204.
60. Miller JW, Green R, Ramos MI, et al. Homocysteine and cognitive function in the Sacramento Area Latino Study on Aging. Am J Clin Nutr 2003;78:441–7.

61. Elias MF, Sullivan LM, D'Agostino RB, et al. Homocysteine and cognitive performance in the Framingham offspring study: age is important. Am J Epidemiol 2005;162:644–53.
62. Prins ND, Den Heijer T, Hofman A, et al. Homocysteine and cognitive function in the elderly: the Rotterdam Scan Study. Neurology 2002;59:1375–80.
63. Deschaintre Y, Richard F, Leys D, et al. Treatment of vascular risk factors is associated with slower decline of Alzheimer disease. Neurology 2009;73(9):674–80.
64. Gorelick PB, Scuteri A, Black SE, et al. Vascular contributions to cognitive impairment and dementia: a statement for healthcare professionals for the American Heart Association/American Stroke Association. Stroke 2011;42:2672–713.
65. Weinstein AM, Barton C, Ross L, et al. Treatment practices of mild cognitive impairment in California Alzheimer's disease centers. J Am Geriatr Soc 2009;57(4):686–90.
66. Raschetti R, Albanese E, Vanacore N, et al. Cholinesterase inhibitors in mild cognitive impairment: a systematic review of randomized trials. PLoS Med 2007;4(11):e338.
67. Feldman HH, Ferris S, Winblad B, et al. Effect of rivastigmine on delay to diagnosis of Alzheimer's disease from mild cognitive impairment: the index study. Lancet Neurol 2007;6(6):501–12.
68. Petersen RC, Thomas RG, Grundman M, et al. Vitamin E and donepezil for the treatment of mild cognitive impairment. N Engl J Med 2005;352(23):2379–88.
69. Diniz BS, Pinto JA Jr, Gonzaga ML, et al. To treat or not to treat? A meta-analysis of the use of cholinesterase inhibitors in mild cognitive impairment for delaying progression to Alzheimer's disease. Eur Arch Psychiatry Clin Neurosci 2009;259(4):248–56.
70. Sano M, Ernesto C, Thomas RG, et al. A controlled trial of selegiline, alpha-tocopherol, or both as treatment for Alzheimer's disease. N Engl J Med 1997;336(17):1216–22.
71. McShane R, Areosa SA, Minakaran N. Memantine for dementia. Cochrane Database Syst Rev 2006;(2):CD003154. http://dx.doi.org/10.1002/14651858. CD003154.pub5.
72. Winblad B, Jelic V. Treating the full spectrum of dementia with memantine. Int J Geriatr Psychiatry 2003;18(S1):S41–6.
73. Ferris S, Schneider L, Farmer M, et al. A double-blind, placebo-controlled trial of memantine in age-associated memory impairment (memantine in AAMI). Int J Geriatr Psychiatry 2007;22(5):448–55.
74. Posadski P, Ernst E, Lee MS. Complementary and alternative medicine for Alzheimer's disease: an overview of systematic reviews. Focus Altern Complement Ther 2012;17(4):186–91.
75. Resnick B, Pacala JT. 2012 Beers criteria. J Am Geriatr Soc 2012;60:612–3.
76. McGuinness B, O'Hare J, Craig D, et al. Cochrane review on 'Statins for the treatment of dementia'. Int J Geriatr Psychiatry 2013;28(2):119–26. http://dx.doi.org/10.1002/gps.3797.
77. Van der Most PJ, Dolga AM, Nijholt IM, et al. Statins: mechanisms of neuroprotection. Prog Neurobiol 2009;88(1):64–75.
78. Sparks DL. Statins in the treatment of Alzheimer disease. Nat Rev Neurol 2011;7:662–3. http://dx.doi.org/10.1038/nrneurol.2011.165.
79. Padala KP, Padala PR, McNeilly DP, et al. The effect of HMG-COA reductase inhibitors on cognition in patients with Alzheimer's dementia: a prospective

withdrawal and rechallenge pilot study. Am J Geriatr Pharmacother 2012;10(5): 296–302.

80. Evans MA, Golomb BA. Statin-associated adverse cognitive effects: survey results from 171 patients. Pharmacotherapy 2009;29(7):800–11.

81. Wouter Jukema J, Cannon CP, De Craen AJ, et al. The controversies of Statin therapy: weighing the evidence. J Am Coll Cardiol 2012;60(10):875–81.

82. Corsentino EA, Sawyer K, Sachs-Ericsson N, et al. Depressive symptoms moderate the influence of apolipoprotein epsilon4 allele on cognitive decline in a sample of community dwelling older adults. Am J Geriatr Psychiatry 2009; 17(2):155–65.

83. Boyle PA, Buchman AS, Barnes L, et al. Effect of a purpose in life on risk of incident Alzheimer disease and mild cognitive impairment in community-dwelling older persons. Arch Gen Psychiatry 2010;67(3):304–10.

84. Fratiglioni L, Paillard-Borg S, Winblad B. An active and socially integrated lifestyle in late life might protect against dementia. Lancet Neurol 2004;3(6):343–53.

85. Bennett DA, Schneider JA, Tang Y, et al. The effect of social networks on the relation between Alzheimer's disease pathology and level of cognitive function in old people: a longitudinal cohort study. Lancet Neurol 2006;5(5): 406–12.

86. Lindfors P, Lundberg U. Is low cortisol level an indicator of positive health? Stress Health 2002;18:153–60.

87. Friedman EM, Hayney M, Love GD, et al. Plasma interleukin-6 and soluble il-6 receptors are associated with psychological well-being in aging women. Health Psychol 2007;26(3):305–13.

88. Willis SL, Tennstedt SL, Marsiske M, et al. Long term effects of cognitive training on everyday functional outcomes in older adults. JAMA 2006;296(23):2805–14.

89. Kurz A, Pohl C, Ramsenthaler M, et al. Cognitive rehabilitation in patients with mild cognitive impairment. Int J Geriatr Psychiatry 2009;24:163–8.

90. Ball K, Berch DB, Helmers KF, et al, Advanced Cognitive Training for Independent and Vital Elderly Study Group. Effects of cognitive training interventions with older adults: a randomized controlled trial. JAMA 2002;288:2271–81.

91. Kurz AF, Leucht S, Lautenschlager NT. The clinical significance of cognition-focused interventions for cognitively impaired older adults: a systematic review of randomized controlled trials. Int Psychogeriatr 2011;1(1):1–12.

92. Belleville S. Cognitive training for persons with mild cognitive impairment. Int Psychogeriatr 2008;20:57–66.

93. Petersen RC, Morris JC. Mild cognitive impairment as a clinical entity and treatment target. Arch Neurol 2005;62:1160–3.

94. Bandura A. Self-efficacy: the exercise of control. New York: WH Freeman; 1997.

95. Yalom ID. The theory and practice of group psychotherapy. 4th edition. New York: Basic Books; 1995.

96. Clay OJ, Wadley VG, Edwards J, et al. The useful field of view as a predictor of driving performance in older adults: a cumulative meta-analysis. Optom Vis Sci 2005;82:724–31.

97. Anstey KJ, Windsor TD, Luszcz MA, et al. Predicting driving cessation over 5 years in older adults: psychological well-being and cognitive competence are stronger predictors than physical health. J Am Geriatr Soc 2006;54: 121–6.

98. Ackerman MA, Edwards JD, Ross LA, et al. Examination of cognitive and instrumental functional performance as indicators for driving cessation risk across 3 years. Gerontologist 2008;48:802–10.

99. Edwards JD, Ross LA, Ackerman M, et al. Longitudinal predictors of driving cessation among older adults from the ACTIVE clinical trial. J Gerontol B Psychol Sci Soc Sci 2008;63:P6–12.

100. Edwards JD, Myers C, Ross LA, et al. The longitudinal impact of cognitive speed of processing training on driving mobility. Gerontologist 2009;49(4): 485–94.

101. Teng E, Becker BW, Woo E, et al. Subtle deficits in instrumental activities of daily living in subtypes of mild cognitive impairment. Dement Geriatr Cogn Disord 2010;30(3):189–97.

102. Goldberg TE, Koppel J, Keehlisen L, et al. Performance-based measures of everyday function in mild cognitive impairment. Am J Psychiatry 2010;167(7): 845–53.

103. Hughes TF, Chang CC, Bilt JV, et al. Mild cognitive deficits and everyday functioning among older adults in the community: the Monongahela-Youghiogheny Healthy Aging Team study. Am J Geriatr Psychiatry 2012;20:836–44.

104. Bangen KJ, Jak AJ, Schiehser DM, et al. Complex activities of daily living vary by mild cognitive impairment subtype. J Int Neuropsychol Soc 2010;16(4): 630–9.

105. Scogin F, Shah A. Making evidence-based psychological treatments work with older adults. Washington, DC: American Psychological Association; 2012.

106. Kramer AF, Bherer L, Colcombe SJ, et al. Environmental influences on cognitive and brain plasticity during aging. J Gerontol A Biol Sci Med Sci 2004;59(9): M940–57.

107. Spirduso WW. Reaction and movement time as a function of age and physical activity level. J Gerontol 1975;30:18–23.

108. Colcombe S, Kramer AF. Fitness effects on the cognitive function of older adults: a meta analytic study. Psychol Sci 2003;14:125–30.

109. Marmeleira JF, Godinho MB, Fernandes OM. The effects of an exercise program on several abilities associated with driving performance in older adults. Accid Anal Prev 2009;41(1):90–7.

110. Morris MC, Evans DA, Tangney CC, et al. Fish consumption and cognitive decline with age in a large community study. Arch Neurol 2005;62(12):1849–53.

111. Fotuhi M, Mohassel P, Yaffe K. Fish consumption, long-chain omega-3 fatty acids and risk of cognitive decline or Alzheimer disease: a complex association. Nat Clin Pract Neurol 2009;5(3):140–52.

112. Scarmeas N, Stern Y, Mayeux R, et al. Mediterranean diet and mild cognitive impairment. Arch Neurol 2009;66:216–25.

113. Piazza-Gardner AK, Gaffud TJ, Barry AE. The impact of alcohol on Alzheimer's disease: a systematic review. Aging Ment Health 2012;17(2):133–46.

114. Solfrizzi V, D'Introno A, Colacicco AM, et al. Alcohol consumption, mild cognitive impairment, and progression to dementia. Neurology 2007;68(21):1790–9.

115. Carpenter BD, Xiong C, Porensky EK, et al. Reaction to a dementia diagnosis in individuals with Alzheimer's disease and mild cognitive impairment. J Am Geriatr Soc 2008;56:405–12.

116. West RL, Bagwell DK, Dark-Freudeman A. Self-efficacy and memory aging: the impact of a memory intervention based on self-efficacy. Aging Neuropsychol Cognit 2007;15:302–29.

117. Bensadon BA. Self-efficacy and memory aging [master's thesis]. Gainesville (FL): University of Florida; 2007.

118. Bensadon BA. Memory self-efficacy and stereotype effects in aging [dissertation]. Gainesville (FL): University of Florida; 2010.

119. Matthews FE, Stephan BC, Bond J, et al, Medical Research Council Cognitive Function and Ageing Study. Operationalization of mild cognitive impairment: a graphical approach. PLoS Med 2007;4:1615–9.

120. Stephan BC, Matthews FE, McKeith IG, et al, Medical Research Council Cognitive Function and Ageing Study. Early cognitive change in the general population: how do different definitions work? J Am Geriatr Soc 2007;55: 1534–40.

121. Stephan BC, Matthews FE, Khaw KT, et al. Beyond mild cognitive impairment: vascular cognitive impairment, no dementia (VCIND). Alzheimers Res Ther 2009;1(1):4.

122. Kane KD, Yochim BP, Lichtenberg PA. Depressive symptoms and cognitive impairment predict all-cause mortality in long-term care residents. Psychol Aging 2010;25(2):446–52.

123. World Health Organization. Mental health: suicide prevention. World Health Organization Web site. 2013. Available at: http://www.who.int/mental_health/prevention/suicide/suicideprevent/en/. Accessed January 8, 2013.

124. Centers for Disease Control and Prevention. Web-based injury and reporting system. Injury prevention and control: data and statistics (WISQARS). Centers for Disease Control Web site. 2013. Available at: http://www.cdc.gov/injury/wisqars/index.html. Accessed January 8, 2013.

125. Kaplan MS, McFarland BH, Huguet N, et al. Suicide risk and precipitating circumstances among young, middle-aged, and older male veterans. Am J Public Health 2012;102(1):S131–7.

126. Kellermann AL, Rivara FP. Silencing the science on gun research. JAMA 2012; 21:E1–2.

127. Fiske A, Wetherell JL, Gatz M. Depression in older adults. Annu Rev Clin Psychol 2009;5:363–89.

128. Conwell Y, Brent D. Suicide and aging I: patterns of psychiatric diagnosis. In: Pearson JL, Conwell Y, editors. Suicide: international perspectives. New York: Springer; 1996. p. 15–30.

129. McMillan D, Gilbody S, Beresford E, et al. Can we predict suicide and non-fatal self-harm with the Beck Hopelessness Scale? A meta-analysis. Psychol Med 2007;37:769–78.

130. Joiner TE, Sachs-Ericsson NJ, Wingate LR, et al. Perceived burdensomeness and suicidality: two studies on the suicide notes of those attempting and those completing suicide. J Soc Clin Psychol 2002;21:531–45.

131. Luoma JB, Martin CE, Pearson JL. Contact with mental health and primary care providers before suicide: a review of the evidence. Am J Psychiatry 2002;159: 909–16.

132. Lachs MS, Pillemer K. Abuse and neglect of elderly persons. N Engl J Med 1995;332(7):437–43.

133. Kroenke K, Spitzer RL, Williams JB. The PHQ-9: validity of a brief depression severity measure. J Gen Intern Med 2001;16(9):606–13.

134. Odenheimer GL, Hunt L. Functional assessment in geriatric neurology. In: Albert ML, Knoefel JE, editors. Clinical neurology of aging. 3rd edition. USA: Oxford University Press; 2011. p. 149–56.

135. Vance DE, Roenker DL, Cissell GM, et al. Predictors of driving exposure and avoidance in a field study of older drivers from the state of Maryland. Accid Anal Prev 2006;38(4):823–31.

136. Lucas-Blaustein MJ, Filipp L, Dungan C, et al. Driving in patients with dementia. J Am Geriatr Soc 1988;36:1087–91.

137. Friedland RP, Koss E, Kumar A, et al. Motor vehicle crashes in dementia of the Alzheimer type. Ann Neurol 1988;24:782–6.
138. Ball KK, Roenker DL, Wadley VG, et al. Can high-risk older drivers be identified through performance-based measures in a Department of Motor Vehicles setting? J Am Geriatr Soc 2006;54(1):77–84.
139. Ross LA, Clay OJ, Edwards JD, et al. Do older drivers at risk for crashes modify their driving over time? J Gerontol B Psychol Sci Soc Sci 2009; 64B(2):163–70.
140. Carr DB, Ott BR. The older adult driver with cognitive impairment: it's a very frustrating life. JAMA 2000;303(16):1632–41.
141. Wadley VG, Okonkwo O, Crow M, et al. Mild cognitive impairment and everyday function: an investigation of driving performance. J Geriatr Psychiatry Neurol 2009;22(2):87–94.
142. Francis V, Korsch BM, Morris MJ. Gaps in doctor-patient communication–patients' response to medical advice. N Engl J Med 1969;280:535–40.
143. Hall JA, Roter DL, Katz NR. Meta-analysis of correlates of provider behavior in medical encounters. Med Care 1988;26(7):657–75.
144. Roter DL, Hall JA, Merisca R, et al. Effectiveness of interventions to improve patient compliance. Med Care 1998;36(8):1138–61.

Risk Factors for the Progression of Mild Cognitive Impairment to Dementia

Noll L. Campbell, PharmD[a,b,c,d],*, Fred Unverzagt, PhD[e],
Michael A. LaMantia, MD, MPH[b,c,f], Babar A. Khan, MD, MS[b,c,f],
Malaz A. Boustani, MD, MPH[b,c,f]

KEYWORDS

- Mild cognitive impairment • Dementia • Risk factors • Genetics • Biomarkers

KEY POINTS

- Medial temporal lobe atrophy, total Tau proteins, and $A\beta_{1-42}$ have been used as markers of disease processes that improve the identification of preclinical cognitive impairment.
- Modifiable risk factors, such as hypertension, diabetes, and depression, represent potential areas for therapeutic interventions to minimize the progression of mild cognitive impairment (MCI).
- Future interventions targeting cardiovascular and other clinical interventions must consider the complexities of medication management in attempts to reduce the progression of MCI to dementia.

INTRODUCTION

As identified in previously published articles, including those published in this issue, the detection of early cognitive impairment among older adult populations is worthy of diagnostic and clinical recognition. Several definitions and classifications have been applied to this form of cognitive impairment over time[1–4] including mild cognitive impairment (MCI),[4–6] cognitive impairment no dementia,[7,8] malignant senescent

Funding Support: This work was supported by grant R01 HS019818-01 from the Agency for Healthcare Research and Quality. The sponsor had no role in the article development.
The authors report no conflicts of interest for this article.
[a] College of Pharmacy, Purdue University, 575 Stadium Mall Drive, West Lafayette, IN 47907, USA; [b] Indiana University Center for Aging Research, 410 West 10th Street, Indianapolis, IN 46202, USA; [c] Regenstrief Institute, Inc, 410 West 10th Street, Indianapolis, IN 46202, USA; [d] Department of Pharmacy, Wishard/Eskenazi Health Services, 1001 West 10th Street, Indianapolis, IN 46202, USA; [e] Department of Psychiatry, Indiana University School of Medicine, 340 West 10th Street, Indianapolis, IN 46202, USA; [f] Department of Medicine, Indiana University School of Medicine, 340 West 10th Street, Indianapolis, IN 46202, USA
* Corresponding author. Department of Pharmacy Practice, Purdue University College of Pharmacy, 410 West 10th Street, Suite 2000, Indianapolis, IN 46202.
E-mail address: campbenl@iupui.edu

forgetfulness,[9] and age-associated cognitive decline.[10] Consistent with current usage this review uses the term MCI, and focuses on progression from MCI to dementia.

Prevalence estimates of MCI among populations of community-dwelling older adults are as high as 22% of those aged 71 years and older,[11] with prevalence rates among older adults cared for in memory care practices estimated at nearly 40%.[12] The likelihood of progression from MCI to any form of dementia has been suggested to occur at a rate 3 to 5 times higher than those with normal cognition,[4,13–15] with an annual rate of progression of 12% in the general population and up to 20% in populations at higher risk.[11] As a transitional stage of early cognitive impairment, much attention has been focused on the identification of modifiable and nonmodifiable risk factors to prevent or delay the progression of MCI to dementia.

Several known risk factors for the development of dementias have been identified, including age, genetic characteristics, lower educational attainment, and various clinical characteristics.[16–20] Among those with MCI, several risk factors influencing the progression to dementia have been identified and are discussed in detail in this clinical review. Early studies aiming to prevent the onset of Alzheimer-type dementia among older adults with amnestic MCI have been reported, including a study using the only approved pharmacologic class in dementia, acetylcholinesterase inhibitors, or vitamin E. The investigators reported that acetylcholinesterase inhibitors did not delay the progression to Alzheimer-type dementia over 3 years, except in those who were carriers of an apolipoprotein ε4 (APOE ε4) allele.[21] A second study evaluating donepezil in reducing the progression of MCI did not show significant improvement in cognition with higher adverse events and dropouts, but did not evaluate for the presence of APOE alleles or the diagnosis of dementia as an outcome.[22] A second prevention study found that cognitive training did not delay the progression from MCI to dementia.[23] Additional studies evaluating potential methods to delay or reduce the likelihood of progression from MCI to dementia have generally found no evidence of support for nonsteroidal anti-inflammatory drugs (NSAIDs) or ginkgo biloba,[24–26] further limiting the potential therapeutic options.

To assist clinicians in understanding factors associated with the progression from MCI to dementia, this article reviews both markers of disease activity and clinical risk factors influencing the progression of MCI to dementia. Biomarkers and imaging characteristics have been extensively studied as pathologic indicators of neurologic disease. The authors first review the validity of biomarkers in monitoring the progression from MCI to dementia. Risk factors for the progression of MCI to dementia are then reviewed, and categorized as modifiable and nonmodifiable. Modifiable risk factors, such as cardiovascular risk factors, depression, or adverse drug effects, are defined as characteristics that, if manipulated (such as improved success at treatment goals), may modify the risk or rate of progression to dementia. Nonmodifiable risk factors are defined as risk factors that cannot be manipulated, such as demographic or genetic characteristics. Such categorization may provide a platform for future clinical interventions targeting modifiable risk factors to reduce the progression of MCI to dementia.

MARKERS OF DISEASE PROCESS
Imaging

Progressive atrophy of the brain can be detected by structural magnetic resonance imaging (MRI), and has been shown to monitor the disease process in those developing Alzheimer-type dementia.[27–30] Structural MRI has proven sensitivity in monitoring changes with aging,[31–33] and is also sensitive to the detection of a more rapid rate of change as seen when cognitive symptoms progress to dementia.[34] The patterns of change within various regions of the cortex have been shown to have predictive value for progressive cognitive impairment and Alzheimer-type dementia among those with MCI.[35–37] A small study of Italian older adults with MCI found that atrophy of the medial temporal lobe identified on MRI was a better predictor of the progression from MCI to any form of dementia than were baseline neuropsychiatric assessments and demographic characteristics.[38]

White matter lesions (WML) are recognized as areas of higher signal intensity on MRI and are common in older adults, with higher frequencies among those with vascular risk factors.[39–41] Compared with healthy controls, these lesions are progressively more extensive among those with MCI and both vascular and Alzheimer-type dementia.[42,43] A higher severity of lesions has also been identified in those with worse cognitive impairment reported by neuropsychiatric assessment in comparison with healthy controls.[41,44] A recent study by Devine and colleagues[45] evaluated the WML severity and the time to conversion to any form of dementia among a small group of older adults with MCI receiving care in a memory clinic in the United Kingdom. The investigators found no relationship between WML severity and the time to progression to dementia. Age and subtype of dementia were the only independent variables associated with a shorter time to conversion to dementia, noting that more advanced age and the amnestic subtype of MCI progressed to dementia sooner. As Alzheimer-type dementia was the primary type of dementia diagnosed in this group (62%), this result appears to be consistent with a recent review by Debette and Markus[46] suggesting that WML reflect cardiovascular disease burden and are more consistently associated with an increased risk of the progression to vascular or mixed dementias, but not Alzheimer-type dementia. However, a recent article by Brickman and colleagues[47] shows an association between white matter hyperintensities and incident Alzheimer-type dementia in a population without MCI at baseline. The conflicting evidence underscores a lack of accepted opinion in this matter. In addition, a study by Bombois and colleagues[48] also supports the association of imaging with vascular and mixed dementia, noting that increasing amounts of subcortical hyperintensities were only associated with vascular or mixed dementias.

Central and Peripheral Biomarkers

Cerebrospinal fluid (CSF) biomarkers, focusing on detection of Tau proteins and amyloid-β (Aβ) proteins, have also been studied as predictors of the progression of MCI to Alzheimer-type dementia.[49–52] Because of their predictive value, structural MRI and CSF biomarkers have been used as outcome measures to increase trial power and reduce the sample-size burden.[53,54] In addition, biomarkers have been incorporated into recently released recommendations from the National Institute on Aging and the Alzheimer's Association for the recognition of MCI and stratification into diagnostic subtypes of MCI that better describe the risk of progression to Alzheimer-type dementias.[55]

Time to progression of MCI has been evaluated by CSF biomarkers and MRI results in 91 Dutch older adults with MCI who progressed to Alzheimer-type dementia.[56] Predictors of time to progression of MCI to Alzheimer-type dementia included only atrophy of medial temporal lobe (hazard ratio [HR] 2.6, 95% confidence interval [CI] 1.1–6.1; $P = .03$), whereas APOE $\epsilon4$ genotype and Aβ_{1-42} were not associated with time to progression to Alzheimer-type dementia. This result suggests that markers of brain injury (such as Tau proteins or imaging results suggesting progressive neurologic damage), but not pathologic markers (such as Aβ_{1-42}), may better predict the time to progression to Alzheimer-type dementia among older adults with MCI.[56]

Peripheral biomarkers have also been considered, given the challenges in acquiring CSF samples and translating CSF studies to the general population. To date the evaluation of peripheral markers, including various species of cytokines,[57–59] Aβ and other serum proteins,[60–68] and APOE ε isoforms,[69] have not identified clear and reproducible peripheral biomarkers associated with an increased risk of Alzheimer-type dementia. Llano and colleagues[70] recently published on the use of data from the Alzheimer's Disease Neuroimaging (ADNI) project to identify 5 plasma analytes with modest predictive value in differentiating subjects with Alzheimer-type dementia from normal controls (range of sensitivity and specificity 74%–85%). No signature panel was able to adequately predict the progression from MCI to Alzheimer-type dementia within this ADNI population. The investigators recognize that the signature panels have insufficient predictive value independently, but theorize that these groups of markers may have value in the future as part of a multicomponent predictive tool.

A recent study by Choo and colleagues[71] pursued the hypothesis that combinations of biomarkers and imaging results would improve the prediction of progression to Alzheimer-type dementia among Swedish older adults with a diagnosis of MCI. After performing a stepwise multivariate logistic regression analysis for the outcome of Alzheimer-type dementia only, the investigators reported parietal glucose metabolic rate and total Tau proteins predicted the progression from MCI to Alzheimer-type dementia. Although APOE genotype, a known predictor for dementia, did predict progression in univariate models, it did not add further predictive capability to the 2-predictor model in this cohort.

NONMODIFIABLE RISK FACTORS
Genetic Characteristics

Long recognized as a risk factor for Alzheimer-type dementia and even MCI, the APOE ε4 allele has emerged as the most consistent genetic risk factor for the progression of MCI to Alzheimer-type dementia.[72] A meta-analysis published in 2011 included data from 35 studies with more than 6000 subjects to evaluate this and other genetic risk factors.[73] The meta-analysis reports that among those with MCI, carriers of any APOE ε4 allele are more than 2 times as likely to progress to Alzheimer-type dementia (**Table 1**). Homozygotes for the APOE ε4 allele had a 4-fold higher risk of progressing to Alzheimer-type dementia compared with noncarriers. Of note, this review did not include results from the Nun study, which did not find an association between APOE status and the outcome of any dementia.[74] Although the risk of Alzheimer-type dementia was found to be higher, the clinical utility of exclusively using APOE genotype to predict progression to dementia was attenuated by a low sensitivity and specificity (0.53 and 0.67, respectively).[73]

Rodriguez-Rodriguez and colleagues[75] studied the link between 8 genetic variants with the risk of progression to Alzheimer-type dementia or with the speed of progression to Alzheimer-type dementia. Among 297 patients seen in a Spanish neurology clinic with a diagnosis of MCI, only 2 genetic variants had an impact on the progression to Alzheimer-type dementia. As expected, the APOE ε4 allele more than quadrupled the risk of progression to Alzheimer-type dementia ($P<.001$). Carriers of the clusterin (CLU) T-allele had a lower risk of conversion to Alzheimer-type dementia than noncarriers of the T-allele. With respect to speed of progression, APOE was the only individual genetic predictor of a more rapid progression (HR 1.77, 95% CI 1.05–2.97; $P = .030$). In addition, the investigators reported that carriers of at least 6 non-APOE genetic variants had a 2-fold increased risk of more rapid progression to Alzheimer-type dementia.

Subtype of MCI

The National Institute on Aging and Alzheimer's Association recently released recommendations for the stratification of MCI categories in the context of the likelihood of progression to Alzheimer-type dementia.[55] Categorization into such groups is based on neuroimaging (such as atrophy of medial temporal lobe) and biomarkers (such as Tau proteins and $A\beta_{1-42}$). Four categories are proposed: those with high likelihood to progress to Alzheimer-type dementia, intermediate likelihood, unlikely, and a core group with conflicting results (**Table 2**). Two studies validated these categories using different populations enrolled either in the ADNI study[76] or the Alzheimer's Disease Research Center or Mayo Clinic Study on Aging cohorts.[77] Guo and colleagues[76] found a higher risk of progression to Alzheimer-type dementia when the high-risk group was compared with the core group (HR 2.3, 95% CI 1.4–3.9; P = .002). Jack and colleagues[77] used the criteria to classify preclinical disease (among those with normal cognition), to improve the understanding of the disease process and promote the optimal intervention point to minimize future disease progression. However, because categorical definitions for early disease processes and MCI subtypes has been recently released, the majority of categorization schemes have defined MCI subtypes as amnestic or nonamnestic and single-domain or multi-domain characteristics.

A subtype of MCI was suggested to identify the possible neurologic abnormality to describe the progression to different dementias in a study of older adults with MCI cared for in a California Alzheimer disease center.[13] After a mean follow-up time of 3 years, 65% progressed to any form of dementia; those with amnestic forms of MCI were more likely to progress to Alzheimer-type dementia, whereas nonamnestic forms were more likely to progress to vascular or frontotemporal dementia. Similarly, in a population of 60 Italian older adults followed for a mean of 4 years, any type of MCI increased the risk for any dementia (HR 3.02, 95% CI 1.86–4.89) as well as Alzheimer-type dementia (HR 3.21, 95% CI 1.77–5.81), but not vascular dementia. This risk appeared to be attributable to the risk of amnestic MCI in the progression to any dementia (see **Table 1**); and, interestingly, the risk of progression to any dementia was no different among those with nonamnestic MCI and those without MCI. However, it must be noted that the sample size with nonamnestic MCI was too small to draw conclusions.[78]

Zhou and colleagues[79] recently highlighted predictors of progression to dementia among the ADNI cohort with MCI by focusing on demographic, genetic, imaging, and cognitive assessments conducted at baseline. The investigators conducted Cox proportional hazard regression models to identify variables increasing the risk of progression to dementia, and further characterized these risks into survival trees. Stepwise Cox regression analysis determined the Alzheimer's Disease Assessment Scale with 13 items (ADAS13) and logical memory with delayed recall as the 2 tests most frequently identifying abnormal results. Alzheimer-type dementia developed in the entire cohort at a rate of 5.6% at 12 months and 58.1% at 48 months. Considering a combination of baseline ADAS13 scores greater than 15.67 and Clinical Dementia Rating scale sum of boxes (CDR-sob) scores greater than 1.5 yielded an incident Alzheimer-type dementia rate of 12.9% at 12 months and 92.7% at 48 months. Using the ADAS13 as the first categorization method, the strength of this predictive risk stratification was similar when either baseline battery tests or imaging measures of cortical thickness of the right inferior temporal lobe were used, all with a similar c-index of 0.68. Although a promising lead, it must be restated that the population included in the ADNI cohort may have limited translation to populations cared for in many clinical settings.

Table 1
Factors modifying the progression from MCI to any form of dementia reported in at least one published study

Authors,[Ref.] Year	Sample Size and Cohort Definition	Variable	Outcome Definition	Hazard Ratio (95% CI)	Comment
Genetics					
Elias-Sonnenschein et al,[73] 2011	Meta-analysis of 35 studies including >6000 subjects	APOE ε4	Alzheimer-type dementia	2.29 (1.88–2.80)	Progression to Alzheimer-type dementia in homozygotes: 3.94 (2.09–7.33)
Rodriguez-Rodriguez et al,[75] 2012	288 Spanish older adults with MCI	APOE ε4, CLU	Alzheimer-type dementia	APOE ε4: 4.56 (2.23–9.38) CLU: 0.25 (0.07–0.84)	Carriers of at least 6 genetic risk factors increased the risk of more rapid progression (HR 1.89, 95% CI 1.01–3.56)
Tyas et al,[74] 2007	470 subjects from the Nun study	APOE ε4	Any dementia	1.12 (0.60–2.08)	Age was the only predictor for the progression of MCI to dementia
MCI Subtype					
Ravaglia et al,[78] 2008	60 Italian older adults with MCI; 27 with at least memory-domain MCI	MCI with at least memory impairment	Any dementia or Alzheimer-type dementia	Any: 4.78 (2.83–8.07) Alzheimer: 5.92 (3.30–10.91)	No difference in progression to dementia between those with nonamnestic MCI and those without MCI
Zhou et al,[79] 2012	397 older adults with MCI from the ADNI cohort	ADAS13 and CDR-sob scores	Alzheimer-type dementia	6.9 (4.3–11.0)	High-risk groups included those with ADAS13 >15.67 and CDR-sob >1.5

Study	Sample	Predictor	Outcome	Results (HR/OR)	Findings
Koepsell and Monsell,[80] 2012	3020 American older adults with MCI	Nonamnestic single domain, MMSE and CDR scores, and FAQ score	Reversion to normal cognition	Nonamnestic single domain: 1.75 (1.29–2.38) MMSE: 1.21 (1.12–1.30) CDR-sob: 0.66 (0.57–0.77) FAQ $\geq$1: 0.72 (0.56–0.94)	After 1 year of follow-up, 16% reverted to normal cognition and 20% progressed to dementia. Categorical comparison groups were amnestic single-domain, FAQ score of 0, and APOE ε4 noncarriers
Yaffe et al,[13] 2006	305 American older adults with MCI	MCI subtype: reference group was amnestic MCI	Any dementia	Single, nonamnestic: 0.60 (0.35–1.05) Multidomain MCI: 0.71 (0.44–1.14)	MCI subtype predicted dementia type: amnestic MCI more likely to develop Alzheimer-type dementia; single nonamnestic MCI predicted FTD
Comorbidity					
Solfrizzi et al,[91] 2011	121 Italian older adults	Metabolic syndrome	Any dementia	7.80 (1.29–47.20)	Metabolic syndrome did not increase risk of incident MCI
Li et al,[92] 2012	257 Chinese older adults with MCI	MRI, CTA, and clinical characteristics	Any dementia	Diabetes: 2.39 (1.07–5.33) WMC: 0.06 (0.02–0.20) Carotid stenosis: 159.06 (4.57–5537.67)	Similar risk of progression to Alzheimer-type dementia
Clerici et al,[93] 2012	245 Italian older adults receiving care in a memory disorders clinic	MRI and clinical characteristics	Any or Alzheimer-type dementias	Combination of $\geq$1 deep WML and HIS $\geq$4: 3.5 (1.6–7.4)	Similar result for the association with Alzheimer-type dementia

(continued on next page)

Table 1
(continued)

Authors,[Ref.] Year	Sample Size and Cohort Definition	Variable	Outcome Definition	Hazard Ratio (95% CI)	Comment
Xu et al,[98] 2010	302 Swedish older adults with MCI	Diabetes or prediabetes	Any or Alzheimer-type dementias	3.89 (1.69–8.32)	Similar risk of Alzheimer-type as with any dementia. Markers of disease control not considered
DeCarli et al,[95] 2004	52 American adults with MCI visiting a memory clinic	Vascular risk factors	Alzheimer-type dementia (by CDR-sob score)	Not significantly different, no HR reported	Poor memory and executive function increased the risk of progression to Alzheimer-type dementia
Li et al,[99] 2011	837 Chinese older adults with MCI	Vascular risk factors	Alzheimer-type dementia	Treatment reduced Alzheimer dementia	Treatment of more risk factors reduced the risk more than treatment of fewer risk factors
Ravaglia et al,[94] 2006	165 Italian older adults with MCI	Vascular risk factors	Any dementia	Diastolic blood pressure: 0.52 (0.32–0.84) Atrial fibrillation: 4.94 (1.89–12.88)	Small number of subjects with atrial fibrillation may limit interpretation. Hypertension not associated with dementia, but diastolic pressure appears protective

Bettermann et al,[101] 2012	482 American older adults with MCI	Statin use	All-cause and Alzheimer-type dementia	No difference between users and nonusers	Statin use reduced the risk of incident dementia in cognitively normal subjects
Neuropsychiatric Symptoms					
Richard et al,[109] 2012	320 older adults from Manhattan, NY, USA	CES-D ≥4	Any dementia	1.8 (1.0–3.1)	Nonsignificant increase in risk of Alzheimer-type dementia
Richard et al,[105] 2012	397 older adults from ADNI	GDS-15—3-item Apathy score	Alzheimer-type dementia	1.85 (1.09–3.15)	Effect only significant in those without depression. A GDS score of ≥6 was an exclusion for the ADNI study
Modrego and Ferrandez,[106] 2004	45 Italian older adults with MCI	Depression (GDS and structured interview)	Alzheimer-type dementia	2.6 (1.8–3.6)	
Palmer et al,[107] 2007	47 Swedish older adults with MCI	Comprehensive Psychopathological Rating Scale	Alzheimer-type dementia	1.8 (1.2–2.7)	Depressed mood increased risk of progression to Alzheimer in cognitively normal subjects
Reynolds et al,[108] 2011	57 American older adults with MCI and depression	Antidepressants with or without donepezil	Any dementia	NR; Reduced rate of progression to dementia (10% vs 33%)	Higher risk of recurrent depression (likelihood ratio: 4.91; $P = .03$)

Abbreviations: ADAS13, Alzheimer's Disease Assessment Scale with 13 items; ADNI, Alzheimer's Disease Neuroimaging project; APOE, apolipoprotein; CDR-sob, Clinical Dementia Rating scale sum of boxes; CES-D, Center for Epidemiological Studies Depression; CI, confidence interval; CLU, clusterin; CTA, computed tomographic angiography; FAQ, Functional Activities Questionnaire; FTD, frontotemporal dementia; GDS, Global Deterioration Scale; HIS, Hachinski Ischemic Score; MCI, mild cognitive impairment; MMSE, Mini-Mental Status Examination; MRI, magnetic resonance imaging; MTL, medial temporal lobe; NR, not reported; WML, white matter lesions.

Table 2
Risk stratification of MCI subtypes as defined by the NIA-AA

Core Criteria: Apply to All	MCI Subtype	Biomarker Indicator	
		Neuronal Injury Result	Imaging Result
1. Complaint of change in cognitive function	MCI Unlikely	Negative	Negative
	MCI Core	Untested/indeterminate	Untested/indeterminate
2. Impairment in more than 1 cognitive domain	MCI Intermediate	Untested/indeterminate	Positive
		Positive	Untested/indeterminate
3. No decline in function	MCI High	Positive	Positive
4. Not dementia			

Abbreviations: MCI, mild cognitive impairment; NIA-AA, National Institute on Aging–Alzheimer's Association.

Adapted from Albert MS, DeKosky ST, Dickson D, et al. The diagnosis of mild cognitive impairment due to Alzheimer's disease: recommendations from the National Institute on Aging-Alzheimer's Association workgroups on diagnostic guidelines for Alzheimer's disease. Alzheimers Dement 2011;7(3):270–9.

In an alternative and complementary approach, Koepsell and Monsell[80] pursued this research question with the objective of identifying predictors of the reversion from MCI to normal cognitive function. The investigators used a cohort of approximately 3000 subjects from the National Alzheimer's Coordinating Center who were at least 65 years old and diagnosed with MCI. After a follow-up period of approximately 1 year, 5 risk factors predicting reversion from MCI to normal cognition were identified: higher baseline Mini-Mental State Examination (MMSE) scores, lower CDR-sob scores, fewer functional impairments, nonamnestic single-domain subtype of MCI, and a lack of APOE ε4 genotype. Of note, these results did not incorporate clinical factors such as burden of vascular disease, and categorized normal cognition as either normal or "impaired but not MCI" as the outcome measure, stating that categorization across multiple centers used each term with variable frequencies. However, the investigators also identified a trend among those patients with MCI who reverted to normal cognitive function that suggests they were more likely to transition back to MCI or to dementia than those cognitively normal at baseline.[80]

MODIFIABLE RISK FACTORS
Comorbidity and Other Clinical Characteristics

Chronic comorbid disease such as coronary heart disease and hypertension are common in older adults who develop cognitive impairment,[81,82] often requiring the use of several medications to reach therapeutic goals. It has been documented that ambulatory older adults use an average of 11 medications per day and that 74% combine prescription medications and dietary supplements.[83,84] Incident cognitive impairment has been suggested to be less likely in those using medications to control for vascular risk factors[85–89]; however, other medications may result in adverse cognitive outcomes, such as MCI, and represent a potentially reversible risk factor.

A descriptive analysis of a population with cognitive impairment (either MCI or dementia) from the Cache County study suggests that those with cognitive impairment have a more severe burden of comorbid disease than those without cognitive impairment.[90] Vascular disease has been considered the most likely comorbidity to cause a more rapid progression of cognitive impairment. One study involving approximately

500 older adults from a Midwestern Alzheimer disease center evaluated risk factors for progression from MCI to dementia. Using a Markov chain model to assess the transition from one cognitive state to another, the investigators did not find an influence of demographic, genetic, or education on the progression to dementia, but rather found that a baseline history of hypertension reduced the likelihood of progression to dementia. This population was largely Caucasian and educated, possibly indicating a higher likelihood of adherence to medications to control hypertension and reduce the burden of vascular disease.

Investigators from the Italian Longitudinal Study in Aging focused an analysis of their population-based database on the relationship of metabolic syndrome with the progression of MCI to dementia.[91] Metabolic syndrome is recognized by the presence of at least 3 of the following features: abdominal obesity (measured by waist circumference), elevated plasma triglyceride levels of at least 150 mg/dL, low high-density lipoprotein cholesterol (<40 mg/dL for men and <50 mg/dL for women), high blood pressure ($\geq$130/$\geq$85 mm Hg), or use of antihypertensive treatment. The study observed approximately 2100 patients over a mean of 3.5 years, only 121 of whom had MCI. Multivariate models adjusting for several potential demographic and cardiovascular confounders revealed a higher risk of progression to any dementia among those with metabolic syndrome. Within this same population, interestingly no relationship between metabolic syndrome and incident MCI was identified.

A prospective study of 257 Chinese older adults with MCI was conducted to identify risk factors for the progression of cognitive decline (evaluated by MMSE score), progression from MCI to any dementia, and progression from MCI to Alzheimer-type dementia.[92] The investigators considered vascular risk factors of diabetes, hypertension, hyperlipidemia, and tobacco and alcohol use over a 3-year observation period. MRI and computed tomographic angiography (CTA) were used to identify changes in white matter and degree of cerebral arteriostenosis. Considering all clinical variables and imaging results, diabetes, baseline severity of white matter change, and carotid stenosis were robust predictors for each outcome, including any dementia and Alzheimer-type dementia. The investigators evaluated the impact of antihypertensive use and oral hypoglycemic or insulin use, and found no association with the progression to dementia.[92] Such results suggest that vascular risk factors resulting in chronic cerebral hypoperfusion have a negative impact on cognitive function and may advance the progression to any form of dementia.

A similar study conducted in an Italian population of community-dwelling older adults with a diagnosis of MCI followed 245 subjects over approximately 2.5 years to evaluate the impact of vascular diseases on the progression of MCI to dementia.[93] Vascular diseases were recognized by the Hachinski Ischemic Score and the Framingham Stroke Risk Profile. The Hachinksi score is a marker of existing cerebrovascular disease, whereas the Framingham Stroke Risk Profile is a marker of future cerebrovascular disease risk. The investigators also considered the presence of APOE ε4, smoking status, and the presence of WML as covariates in the analysis. The results suggest that among the 52% of subjects who progressed to dementia during the observation period, no individual clinical factor or vascular summary score was associated with an increased risk of progression to dementia. However, the combination of Hachinski scores greater than 4 with presence of WML near the basal ganglia increased the risk of progression to any form of dementia as well as to Alzheimer-type dementia (HR 3.8, 95% CI 1.2–11.5) after adjusting for age, sex, education, cumulative illness, MMSE, MCI subtype, and APOE genotype. Framingham Stroke Risk Profile was not associated with an increased risk of progression to dementia, either alone or in combination with imaging results.

Other notable studies have evaluated the role of vascular risk factors on the development of dementia, with conflicting results. Results from some observational studies have produced similar results that show no association between individual risk of cardiovascular disease and incident dementia,[13,94–96] whereas others have suggested vascular risk factors may independently increase the risk of progression to dementia.[97–99] In 2004 DeCarli and colleagues[95] reported from a cohort of older adults with MCI and calculated vascular risk through a composite score as the sum of vascular risk factors (up to 6). The investigators also defined Alzheimer-type dementia as a progression from a CDR-sob score of 0.5 to 1.0 or greater. Although limitations in the population as well as the methods are noted, no association between baseline vascular risk factors and progression to Alzheimer-type dementia was identified.

A Swedish longitudinal study on aging reported on the impact of diabetes and prediabetes on the progression from MCI to dementia. Approximately 300 subjects with MCI at baseline were followed for a mean of 3 years. After controlling for age, sex, education, body mass index, genotype, and vascular disorders, the risk of progression to any dementia (see **Table 1**) and Alzheimer-type dementia was increased by a diagnosis of diabetes and prediabetes (HR 4.22, 95% CI 1.57–9.01). Kaplan-Meier survival analysis suggested that diabetes accelerated the time to progression to dementia by an average of 3.2 years. Of note, no risk of incident MCI was identified in older adults with diabetes and normal cognition at baseline.[98]

A recent observational study conducted in a Chinese population over 5 years suggests that vascular risk factors increase the progression of MCI to Alzheimer-type dementia.[99] The investigators report that vascular risk factors (including hypertension, diabetes, cerebrovascular disease, and hypercholesterolemia) additively increase the risk of progression to Alzheimer-type dementia, and that treatment of vascular disease was associated with a reduction in the risk of conversion to dementia. Although medication adherence and clinical treatment targets were not assessed, this study gives strong support to interventions aimed at managing vascular risk factors in those with MCI as a method to reduce the progression to dementia. Further support for the treatment of vascular disease in reducing the neuropathology of Alzheimer-type dementia was published in 2009 by Hoffman and colleagues, who used autopsy evidence to show fewer neuritic plaques and neurofibrillary tangles in those with hypertension who received antihypertensive medication than in those not receiving antihypertensive medication.[100]

Contrasting such results, a secondary analysis of the Ginkgo Evaluation in Memory Study described the role of statins on the progression from MCI to dementia in this observational study.[101] Among those with a baseline diagnosis of MCI, statins were found to have no influence on the progression from MCI to all-cause or Alzheimer-type dementia, although statins were shown to reduce incident dementia in the cohort that was cognitively normal at baseline (HR 0.79, 95% CI 0.65–0.96). Though a promising result for incident dementia, this analysis was conducted with self-reported measures of medication exposure, suggesting this association requires further study with more accurate measures of medication exposure as well as control of disease state.

Neuropsychiatric Symptoms

Neuropsychiatric symptoms have been reported in up to 30% of older adults with a diagnosis of MCI.[102] Because neuropsychiatric symptoms have been associated with a worse prognosis in dementia,[103] the relationship between neuropsychiatric symptoms and the risk for progression of MCI to dementia was assessed in a population enrolled from Cache County, Utah.[104] A cohort of 230 older adults diagnosed with MCI was evaluated for predictors of progression to any dementia using a cognitive and neuropsychiatric battery (MMSE, Modified MMSE, CDR, and the Neuro-psychiatric Inventory [NPI]). In multivariate regression models controlling for age, education, and APOE status, nighttime behaviors predicted progression to all-cause dementia (HR 1.28, 95% CI 1.08–1.52) and hallucinations predicted progression only to vascular dementia, not all-cause or Alzheimer-type dementia (HR 10.1, 95% CI 1.1–91.1). Overall scores on the NPI suggest that even a minor severity of neuropsy-chiatric symptoms increases the risk of progression to any dementia (HR 1.65, 95% CI 1.01–2.69). Despite the relatively small sample size, this study suggests that further attention to and possibly specific interventions targeting those with neuropsychiatric symptoms may reduce the progression of MCI to dementia.

Other psychiatric symptoms have been evaluated as potential risk factors for the progression of MCI to dementia. Prior work has identified depression and anxiety as 2 risk factors increasing such progression.[105–107] Two of these studies present con-flicting results on the role of depression in the progression of MCI. Whereas both studies assessed depression and anxiety with an outcome of Alzheimer-type demen-tia in populations with amnestic or multidomain MCI, Palmer and colleagues[107] sug-gest that depression alone does not increase the risk of progression to dementia except in those with normal cognition, whereas Modrego and Ferrandez[106] report that the risk of progression is nearly 2-fold in those with depressive symptoms. The 2 studies used different tools to identify depression symptoms, with Modrego using the Geriatric Depression Scale and Palmer identifying symptoms through the Compre-hensive Psychopathological Rating Scale.[106,107] Controversially, the recent study by Peters and colleagues[104] described earlier does not suggest that either depression or anxiety, assessed as domains in the NPI, influenced the progression of MCI to de-mentia. It must be borne in mind that depression and anxiety assessments in the NPI are single-item responses, in comparison with other screening tools assessing 15 to 30 items. However, when Peters and colleagues[104] grouped mood-related domains of depression, anxiety, apathy, and irritability together, no impact on disease progres-sion was revealed. Of note, a recent study by Richard and colleagues[105] found that apathy, but not depressive symptoms, increased the risk of progression from MCI to Alzheimer-type dementia.

The combination of consistent antidepressant treatment (flexible regimen) with or without donepezil in older adults with major depression was recently evaluated. In the cohort with MCI at baseline, adding donepezil to the antidepressant regimen reduced the likelihood of progression to dementia over the 2-year study period; how-ever, this group was also more likely to experience a recurrence of major depression (44% vs 12%, likelihood ratio 4.91; $P = .03$).[108] The investigators appropriately concluded that the potential benefits of adjuvant donepezil and antidepressant therapy require further study, and strong consideration of the risks in the face of the potential benefits.

FUTURE CONSIDERATIONS

Risk stratification based on factors identified in observational studies may offer an opportunity to focus interventions on reducing the risk of incident dementia in those patients at highest risk. As described earlier,[79] existing databases of cohorts with MCI have been used to predict the transition to dementia. **Fig. 1** summarizes the risk factors previously identified to modify the progression from MCI to normal cogni-tion, mixed or vascular dementia, or Alzheimer-type dementia. As a starting point, these results represent promising methods of identifying those populations at highest risk; however, the limitations of such cohorts from the existing literature, often

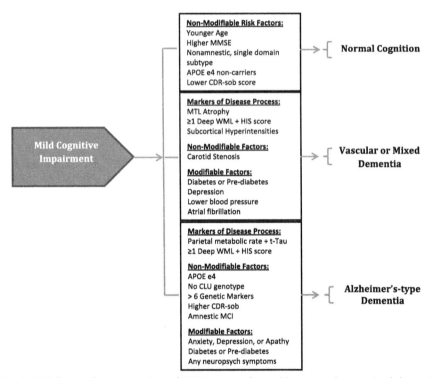

Fig. 1. Risk factors for progression of MCI to normal cognition, vascular or mixed dementia, or Alzheimer-type dementia. APOE, apolipoprotein; CDR-sob, Clinical Dementia Rating scale sum of boxes; CLU, clusterin; HIS, Hachinski Ischemic Score; MMSE, Mini-Mental Status Examination; MCI, mild cognitive impairment; MTL, medial temporal lobe; t-Tau, total Tau protein from cerebrospinal fluid; WML, white matter lesions.

composed of participants involved in research activity, may not represent the population encountered in many clinical environments and reduces the clinical applicability of such results. Similarly, no study has yet focused on interventions such as control of cardiovascular risk factors specifically in those with MCI, making risk-stratification methods applicable to only research environments. To date, studies evaluating the use of acetylcholinesterase inhibitors, NSAIDs, and ginkgo biloba have not yielded results promoting their routine use in clinical practice among those with MCI.

Further evidence is necessary to clarify the impact of comorbid disease, specifically related to the level of disease control, on the progression of MCI to dementia. As noted earlier, there has recently been a significant amount of activity toward understanding the role of comorbid disease on the progression of cognitive impairment. Findings that the treatment of comorbid vascular disease may reduce the likelihood of progression to dementia are promising[22,99]; however, no consideration of the intensity of treatment such as target blood pressure or hemoglobin A_{1c} has been considered. Considering the complexity of medication management and adherence in this population, especially among those experiencing difficulty in executive function, this issue of disease-state control should be pursued with careful attention to risks and benefits of medications. Appropriate methods for assessing medication adherence and monitoring plans that frequently address potential adverse events should be established by clinicians in attempting to control multiple comorbidities in this frail older adult population.

Lastly, although associations between modifiable risk factors, such as hypertension and diabetes, have been suggested, little evidence in the identification of potentially relevant, nonvascular disease states has been pursued, such as oxygen deprivation states of asthma/chronic obstructive pulmonary disease, and severe heart failure. Similarly, certain medications thought to temporarily or permanently impair cognitive function, including anticholinergics, benzodiazepines, and possibly statins, are poorly represented in the existing literature.

SUMMARY

Several risk factors for the progression of cognitive impairment in those diagnosed with MCI have been considered. The variability in results found in the existing literature arises in part from the heterogeneity in populations studied, subtypes of MCI considered, and dementia outcomes evaluated as study end points. Risk factors identified to increase the risk of Alzheimer disease pathology include the presence of deep WML combined with Hachinski Ischemic Scores greater than 4, the presence of APOE ε4 and absence of CLU genotypes, presence of more than 6 genetic markers for Alzheimer-type dementia, amnestic subtype of MCI, psychiatric symptoms of anxiety, depression, or apathy, and presence of diabetes or prediabetes. Risk factors increasing the risk of mixed or vascular dementias include carotid stenosis, diabetes (or prediabetes), depression, low blood pressure, and atrial fibrillation.

From a researcher's perspective, this information is of value as it may improve population selection, design of the intervention, and definition of the outcomes of interest in the quest to minimize the progression of MCI to dementia. Clinicians, patients, and the health care system value this information because it permits a more informed conversation about disease prevention, clinical treatment, and advanced care planning. The risk factors identified thus far represent modifiable and nonmodifiable variables to be incorporated into both research and clinical practice as possible targets for prevention and treatment of progressive cognitive impairment. Given the recognition of common comorbid conditions such as hypertension and diabetes as potentially modifiable risk factors, future management of prevention strategies for the progression of MCI to dementia is likely to fall into the hands of primary care and general practice physicians and mid-level providers.

REFERENCES

1. Ganguli M, Petersen RC. Mild cognitive impairment: challenging issues. Am J Geriatr Psychiatry 2008;16(5):339–42.
2. Winblad B, Palmer K, Kivipelto M, et al. Mild cognitive impairment—beyond controversies, towards a consensus: report of the International Working Group on Mild Cognitive Impairment. J Intern Med 2004;256(3):240–6.
3. Petersen RC. Mild cognitive impairment as a diagnostic entity. J Intern Med 2004;256(3):183–94.
4. Petersen RC, Smith GE, Waring SC, et al. Mild cognitive impairment: clinical characterization and outcome. Arch Neurol 1999;56(3):303–8.
5. Petersen RC, Smith GE, Ivnik RJ, et al. Apolipoprotein E status as a predictor of the development of Alzheimer's disease in memory-impaired individuals. JAMA 1995;273(16):1274–8.
6. Smith G, Petersen RC, Parisi JE, et al. Definition, course, and outcome of mild cognitive impairment. Aging Neuropsychol Cognit 1996;3:131–47.

7. Graham JE, Rockwood K, Beattie BL, et al. Prevalence and severity of cognitive impairment with and without dementia in an elderly population. Lancet 1997; 349(9068):1793–6.

8. Ebly EM, Hogan DB, Parhad IM. Cognitive impairment in the nondemented elderly. Results from the Canadian Study of Health and Aging. Arch Neurol 1995;52(6):612–9.

9. Kral VA. Senescent forgetfulness: benign and malignant. Can Med Assoc J 1962;86:257–60.

10. Levy R. Aging-associated cognitive decline. Working Party of the International Psychogeriatric Association in collaboration with the World Health Organization. Int Psychogeriatr 1994;6(1):63–8.

11. Plassman BL, Langa KM, Fisher GG, et al. Prevalence of cognitive impairment without dementia in the United States. Ann Intern Med 2008;148(6):427–34.

12. Boustani MA, Sachs GA, Alder CA, et al. Implementing innovative models of dementia care: The Healthy Aging Brain Center. Aging Ment Health 2011; 15(1):13–22.

13. Yaffe K, Petersen RC, Lindquist K, et al. Subtype of mild cognitive impairment and progression to dementia and death. Dement Geriatr Cogn Disord 2006; 22(4):312–9.

14. Mitchell AJ, Shiri-Feshki M. Temporal trends in the long term risk of progression of mild cognitive impairment: a pooled analysis. J Neurol Neurosurg Psychiatry 2008;79(12):1386–91.

15. Petersen RC, Roberts RO, Knopman DS, et al. Mild cognitive impairment: ten years later. Arch Neurol 2009;66(12):1447–55.

16. Raffaitin C, Gin H, Empana JP, et al. Metabolic syndrome and risk for incident Alzheimer's disease or vascular dementia: the Three-City Study. Diabetes Care 2009;32(1):169–74.

17. Solfrizzi V, Scafato E, Capurso C, et al. Metabolic syndrome and the risk of vascular dementia: the Italian Longitudinal Study on Ageing. J Neurol Neurosurg Psychiatry 2010;81(4):433–40.

18. Vanhanen M, Koivisto K, Moilanen L, et al. Association of metabolic syndrome with Alzheimer disease: a population-based study. Neurology 2006;67(5): 843–7.

19. Razay G, Vreugdenhil A, Wilcock G. The metabolic syndrome and Alzheimer disease. Arch Neurol 2007;64(1):93–6.

20. Bowler JV. Vascular cognitive impairment. J Neurol Neurosurg Psychiatry 2005; 76(Suppl 5):v35–44.

21. Petersen RC, Thomas RG, Grundman M, et al. Vitamin E and donepezil for the treatment of mild cognitive impairment. N Engl J Med 2005;352(23):2379–88.

22. Doody RS, Ferris SH, Salloway S, et al. Donepezil treatment of patients with MCI: a 48-week randomized, placebo-controlled trial. Neurology 2009;72(18): 1555–61.

23. Unverzagt FW, Guey LT, Jones RN, et al. ACTIVE cognitive training and rates of incident dementia. J Int Neuropsychol Soc 2012;18(4):669–77.

24. Aisen PS, Thal LJ, Ferris SH, et al. Rofecoxib in patients with mild cognitive impairment: further analyses of data from a randomized, double-blind, trial. Curr Alzheimer Res 2008;5(1):73–82.

25. Snitz BE, O'Meara ES, Carlson MC, et al. Ginkgo biloba for preventing cognitive decline in older adults: a randomized trial. JAMA 2009;302(24):2663–70.

26. DeKosky ST, Williamson JD, Fitzpatrick AL, et al. Ginkgo biloba for prevention of dementia: a randomized controlled trial. JAMA 2008;300(19):2253–62.

27. Jack CR Jr, Shiung MM, Weigand SD, et al. Brain atrophy rates predict subsequent clinical conversion in normal elderly and amnestic MCI. Neurology 2005; 65(8):1227–31.

28. Whitwell JL, Shiung MM, Przybelski SA, et al. MRI patterns of atrophy associated with progression to AD in amnestic mild cognitive impairment. Neurology 2008;70(7):512–20.

29. McEvoy LK, Fennema-Notestine C, Roddey JC, et al. Alzheimer disease: quantitative structural neuroimaging for detection and prediction of clinical and structural changes in mild cognitive impairment. Radiology 2009;251(1): 195–205.

30. Bakkour A, Morris JC, Dickerson BC. The cortical signature of prodromal AD: regional thinning predicts mild AD dementia. Neurology 2009;72(12):1048–55.

31. Murphy EA, Holland D, Donohue M, et al. Six-month atrophy in MTL structures is associated with subsequent memory decline in elderly controls. Neuroimage 2010;53(4):1310–7.

32. Becker JA, Hedden T, Carmasin J, et al. Amyloid-beta associated cortical thinning in clinically normal elderly. Ann Neurol 2011;69(6):1032–42.

33. Fjell AM, Walhovd KB, Fennema-Notestine C, et al. One-year brain atrophy evident in healthy aging. J Neurosci 2009;29(48):15223–31.

34. McDonald CR, McEvoy LK, Gharapetian L, et al. Regional rates of neocortical atrophy from normal aging to early Alzheimer disease. Neurology 2009;73(6): 457–65.

35. Saykin AJ, Wishart HA, Rabin LA, et al. Older adults with cognitive complaints show brain atrophy similar to that of amnestic MCI. Neurology 2006;67(5): 834–42.

36. de Leon MJ, Mosconi L, Blennow K, et al. Imaging and CSF studies in the preclinical diagnosis of Alzheimer's disease. Ann N Y Acad Sci 2007;1097:114–45.

37. Tondelli M, Wilcock GK, Nichelli P, et al. Structural MRI changes detectable up to ten years before clinical Alzheimer's disease. Neurobiol Aging 2012;33(4): 825.e25–36.

38. Geroldi C, Rossi R, Calvagna C, et al. Medial temporal atrophy but not memory deficit predicts progression to dementia in patients with mild cognitive impairment. J Neurol Neurosurg Psychiatry 2006;77(11):1219–22.

39. Breteler MM, van Swieten JC, Bots ML, et al. Cerebral white matter lesions, vascular risk factors, and cognitive function in a population-based study: the Rotterdam Study. Neurology 1994;44(7):1246–52.

40. Scarpelli M, Salvolini U, Diamanti L, et al. MRI and pathological examination of post-mortem brains: the problem of white matter high signal areas. Neuroradiology 1994;36(5):393–8.

41. Longstreth WT Jr, Manolio TA, Arnold A, et al. Clinical correlates of white matter findings on cranial magnetic resonance imaging of 3301 elderly people. The Cardiovascular Health Study. Stroke 1996;27(8):1274–82.

42. van der Flier WM, van Straaten EC, Barkhof F, et al. Medial temporal lobe atrophy and white matter hyperintensities are associated with mild cognitive deficits in non-disabled elderly people: the LADIS study. J Neurol Neurosurg Psychiatry 2005;76(11):1497–500.

43. Yoshita M, Fletcher E, Harvey D, et al. Extent and distribution of white matter hyperintensities in normal aging, MCI, and AD. Neurology 2006;67(12):2192–8.

44. de Groot JC, de Leeuw FE, Oudkerk M, et al. Cerebral white matter lesions and subjective cognitive dysfunction: the Rotterdam Scan Study. Neurology 2001; 56(11):1539–45.

45. Devine ME, Fonseca JA, Walker Z. Do cerebral white matter lesions influence the rate of progression from mild cognitive impairment to dementia? Int Psychogeriatr 2013;25(1):120–7.

46. Debette S, Markus HS. The clinical importance of white matter hyperintensities on brain magnetic resonance imaging: systematic review and meta-analysis. BMJ 2010;341:c3666.

47. Brickman AM, Provenzano FA, Muraskin J, et al. Regional white matter hyperintensity volume, not hippocampal atrophy, predicts incident Alzheimer disease in the community. Arch Neurol 2012;69(12):1621–7.

48. Bombois S, Debette S, Bruandet A, et al. Vascular subcortical hyperintensities predict conversion to vascular and mixed dementia in MCI patients. Stroke 2008;39(7):2046–51.

49. Hansson O, Zetterberg H, Buchhave P, et al. Association between CSF biomarkers and incipient Alzheimer's disease in patients with mild cognitive impairment: a follow-up study. Lancet Neurol 2006;5(3):228–34.

50. Mattsson N, Zetterberg H, Hansson O, et al. CSF biomarkers and incipient Alzheimer disease in patients with mild cognitive impairment. JAMA 2009; 302(4):385–93.

51. Mattsson N, Portelius E, Rolstad S, et al. Longitudinal cerebrospinal fluid biomarkers over four years in mild cognitive impairment. J Alzheimers Dis 2012; 30(4):767–78.

52. Fagan AM, Mintun MA, Mach RH, et al. Inverse relation between in vivo amyloid imaging load and cerebrospinal fluid Abeta42 in humans. Ann Neurol 2006; 59(3):512–9.

53. Heister D, Brewer JB, Magda S, et al, Alzheimer's Disease Neuroimaging I. Predicting MCI outcome with clinically available MRI and CSF biomarkers. Neurology 2011;77(17):1619–28.

54. Vos S, van Rossum I, Burns L, et al. Test sequence of CSF and MRI biomarkers for prediction of AD in subjects with MCI. Neurobiol Aging 2012;33(10):2272–81.

55. Albert MS, DeKosky ST, Dickson D, et al. The diagnosis of mild cognitive impairment due to Alzheimer's disease: recommendations from the National Institute on Aging-Alzheimer's Association workgroups on diagnostic guidelines for Alzheimer's disease. Alzheimers Dement 2011;7(3):270–9.

56. van Rossum IA, Visser PJ, Knol DL, et al. Injury markers but not amyloid markers are associated with rapid progression from mild cognitive impairment to dementia in Alzheimer's disease. J Alzheimers Dis 2012;29(2):319–27.

57. Lee KS, Chung JH, Choi TK, et al. Peripheral cytokines and chemokines in Alzheimer's disease. Dement Geriatr Cogn Disord 2009;28(4):281–7.

58. Kamer AR, Craig RG, Pirraglia E, et al. TNF-alpha and antibodies to periodontal bacteria discriminate between Alzheimer's disease patients and normal subjects. J Neuroimmunol 2009;216(1–2):92–7.

59. Bermejo P, Martin-Aragon S, Benedi J, et al. Differences of peripheral inflammatory markers between mild cognitive impairment and Alzheimer's disease. Immunol Lett 2008;117(2):198–202.

60. Seppala TT, Herukka SK, Hanninen T, et al. Plasma Abeta42 and Abeta40 as markers of cognitive change in follow-up: a prospective, longitudinal, population-based cohort study. J Neurol Neurosurg Psychiatry 2010;81(10): 1123–7.

61. Le Bastard N, Leurs J, Blomme W, et al. Plasma amyloid-beta forms in Alzheimer's disease and non-Alzheimer's disease patients. J Alzheimers Dis 2010;21(1):291–301.

62. Lui JK, Laws SM, Li QX, et al. Plasma amyloid-beta as a biomarker in Alzheimer's disease: the AIBL study of aging. J Alzheimers Dis 2010;20(4): 1233–42.
63. Lewczuk P, Kornhuber J, Vanmechelen E, et al. Amyloid beta peptides in plasma in early diagnosis of Alzheimer's disease: a multicenter study with multiplexing. Exp Neurol 2010;223(2):366–70.
64. Blennow K, Zetterberg H. Use of CSF biomarkers in Alzheimer's disease clinical trials. J Nutr Health Aging 2009;13(4):358–61.
65. Kester MI, Verwey NA, van Elk EJ, et al. Evaluation of plasma Abeta40 and Abeta42 as predictors of conversion to Alzheimer's disease in patients with mild cognitive impairment. Neurobiol Aging 2010;31(4):539–40 [author reply: 541].
66. Schupf N, Tang MX, Fukuyama H, et al. Peripheral Abeta subspecies as risk biomarkers of Alzheimer's disease. Proc Natl Acad Sci U S A 2008;105(37): 14052–7.
67. Thambisetty M, Lovestone S. Blood-based biomarkers of Alzheimer's disease: challenging but feasible. Biomark Med 2010;4(1):65–79.
68. Guntert A, Campbell J, Saleem M, et al. Plasma gelsolin is decreased and correlates with rate of decline in Alzheimer's disease. J Alzheimers Dis 2010; 21(2):585–96.
69. Gupta VB, Laws SM, Villemagne VL, et al. Plasma apolipoprotein E and Alzheimer disease risk: the AIBL study of aging. Neurology 2011;76(12):1091–8.
70. Llano DA, Devanarayan V, Simon AJ, et al, The Alzheimer's Disease Neuroimaging Initiative. Evaluation of plasma proteomic data for Alzheimer disease state classification and for the prediction of progression from mild cognitive impairment to Alzheimer disease. Alzheimer Dis Assoc Disord 2013;27(3): 233–43.
71. Choo IH, Ni R, Scholl M, et al. Combination of ^{18}F-FDG PET and cerebrospinal fluid biomarkers as a better predictor of the progression to Alzheimer's disease in mild cognitive impairment patients. J Alzheimers Dis 2013;33(4):929–39.
72. Tschanz JT, Welsh-Bohmer KA, Lyketsos CG, et al. Conversion to dementia from mild cognitive disorder: the Cache County Study. Neurology 2006;67(2):229–34.
73. Elias-Sonnenschein LS, Viechtbauer W, Ramakers IH, et al. Predictive value of APOE-epsilon4 allele for progression from MCI to AD-type dementia: a meta-analysis. J Neurol Neurosurg Psychiatry 2011;82(10):1149–56.
74. Tyas SL, Salazar JC, Snowdon DA, et al. Transitions to mild cognitive impairments, dementia, and death: Findings from the nun study. Am J Epidemiol 2007;165(11):1231–8.
75. Rodriguez-Rodriguez E, Sanchez-Juan P, Vazquez-Higuera JL, et al. Genetic risk score predicting accelerated progression from mild cognitive impairment to Alzheimer's disease. J Neural Transm 2013;120(5):807–12.
76. Guo LH, Alexopoulos P, Eisele T, et al. The National Institute on Aging-Alzheimer's Association research criteria for mild cognitive impairment due to Alzheimer's disease: predicting the outcome. Eur Arch Psychiatry Clin Neurosci 2013;263(4):325–33.
77. Jack CR Jr, Knopman DS, Weigand SD, et al. An operational approach to National Institute on Aging-Alzheimer's Association criteria for preclinical Alzheimer disease. Ann Neurol 2012;71(6):765–75.
78. Ravaglia G, Forti P, Montesi F, et al. Mild cognitive impairment: epidemiology and dementia risk in an elderly Italian population. J Am Geriatr Soc 2008; 56(1):51–8.

79. Zhou B, Nakatani E, Teramukai S, et al, Alzheimer's Disease Neuroimaging I. Risk classification in mild cognitive impairment patients for developing Alzheimer's disease. J Alzheimers Dis 2012;30(2):367–75.

80. Koepsell TD, Monsell SE. Reversion from mild cognitive impairment to normal or near-normal cognition: risk factors and prognosis. Neurology 2012;79(15):1591–8.

81. Campbell NL, Boustani MA, Lane KA, et al. Use of anticholinergics and the risk of cognitive impairment in an African American population. Neurology 2010; 75(2):152–9.

82. Schubert CC, Boustani M, Callahan CM, et al. Comorbidity profile of dementia patients in primary care: are they sicker? J Am Geriatr Soc 2006;54(1):104–9.

83. Murray MD, Young J, Hoke S, et al. Pharmacist intervention to improve medication adherence in heart failure: a randomized trial. Ann Intern Med 2007;146(10): 714–25.

84. Nahin RL, Pecha M, Welmerink DB, et al. Concomitant use of prescription drugs and dietary supplements in ambulatory elderly people. J Am Geriatr Soc 2009; 57(7):1197–205.

85. Murray MD, Lane KA, Gao S, et al. Preservation of cognitive function with antihypertensive medications: a longitudinal analysis of a community-based sample of African Americans. Arch Intern Med 2002;162(18):2090–6.

86. Gorelick PB, Scuteri A, Black SE, et al. Vascular contributions to cognitive impairment and dementia: a statement for healthcare professionals from the American Heart Association/American Stroke Association. Stroke 2011;42(9): 2672–713.

87. Launer LJ, Ross GW, Petrovitch H, et al. Midlife blood pressure and dementia: the Honolulu-Asia aging study. Neurobiol Aging 2000;21(1):49–55.

88. Kivipelto M, Helkala EL, Laakso MP, et al. Midlife vascular risk factors and Alzheimer's disease in later life: longitudinal, population based study. BMJ 2001; 322(7300):1447–51.

89. Hanon O, Berrou JP, Negre-Pages L, et al. Effects of hypertension therapy based on eprosartan on systolic arterial blood pressure and cognitive function: primary results of the Observational Study on Cognitive function and Systolic Blood Pressure Reduction open-label study. J Hypertens 2008;26(8):1642–50.

90. Lyketsos CG, Toone L, Tschanz J, et al. Population-based study of medical co-morbidity in early dementia and "cognitive impairment, no dementia (CIND)": association with functional and cognitive impairment: The Cache County Study. Am J Geriatr Psychiatry 2005;13(8):656–64.

91. Solfrizzi V, Scafato E, Capurso C, et al. Metabolic syndrome, mild cognitive impairment, and progression to dementia. The Italian Longitudinal Study on Aging. Neurobiol Aging 2011;32(11):1932–41.

92. Li L, Wang Y, Yan J, et al. Clinical predictors of cognitive decline in patients with mild cognitive impairment: the Chongqing aging study. J Neurol 2012;259(7): 1303–11.

93. Clerici F, Caracciolo B, Cova I, et al. Does vascular burden contribute to the progression of mild cognitive impairment to dementia? Dement Geriatr Cogn Disord 2012;34(3–4):235–43.

94. Ravaglia G, Forti P, Maioli F, et al. Conversion of mild cognitive impairment to dementia: predictive role of mild cognitive impairment subtypes and vascular risk factors. Dement Geriatr Cogn Disord 2006;21(1):51–8.

95. DeCarli C, Mungas D, Harvey D, et al. Memory impairment, but not cerebrovascular disease, predicts progression of MCI to dementia. Neurology 2004;63(2): 220–7.

96. Wolf H, Ecke GM, Bettin S, et al. Do white matter changes contribute to the subsequent development of dementia in patients with mild cognitive impairment? A longitudinal study. Int J Geriatr Psychiatry 2000;15(9):803–12.

97. Xu WL, Qiu CX, Wahlin A, et al. Diabetes mellitus and risk of dementia in the Kungsholmen project: a 6-year follow-up study. Neurology 2004;63(7):1181–6.

98. Xu W, Caracciolo B, Wang HX, et al. Accelerated progression from mild cognitive impairment to dementia in people with diabetes. Diabetes 2010;59(11): 2928–35.

99. Li J, Wang YJ, Zhang M, et al. Vascular risk factors promote conversion from mild cognitive impairment to Alzheimer disease. Neurology 2011;76(17): 1485–91.

100. Hoffman LB, Schmeidler J, Lesser GT, et al. Less Alzheimer disease neuropathology in medicated hypertensive than nonhypertensive persons. Neurology 2009;72:1720–6.

101. Bettermann K, Arnold AM, Williamson J, et al. Statins, risk of dementia, and cognitive function: secondary analysis of the ginkgo evaluation of memory study. J Stroke Cerebrovasc Dis 2012;21(6):436–44.

102. Peters ME, Rosenberg PB, Steinberg M, et al. Prevalence of neuropsychiatric symptoms in CIND and its subtypes: the Cache County Study. Am J Geriatr Psychiatry 2012;20(5):416–24.

103. Lyketsos CG, Colenda CC, Beck C, et al. Position statement of the American Association for Geriatric Psychiatry regarding principles of care for patients with dementia resulting from Alzheimer disease. Am J Geriatr Psychiatry 2006; 14(7):561–72.

104. Peters ME, Rosenberg PB, Steinberg M, et al. Neuropsychiatric symptoms as risk factors for progression from CIND to Dementia: The Cache County Study. Am J Geriatr Psychiatry 2013. [Epub ahead of print]. http://dx.doi.org/10. 1016/j.jagp.2013.01.049.

105. Richard E, Schmand B, Eikelenboom P, et al. Symptoms of apathy are associated with progression from mild cognitive impairment to Alzheimer's disease in non-depressed subjects. Dement Geriatr Cogn Disord 2012;33(2–3):204–9.

106. Modrego PJ, Ferrandez J. Depression in patients with mild cognitive impairment increases the risk of developing dementia of Alzheimer type: a prospective cohort study. Arch Neurol 2004;61(8):1290–3.

107. Palmer K, Berger AK, Monastero R, et al. Predictors of progression from mild cognitive impairment to Alzheimer disease. Neurology 2007;68(19):1596–602.

108. Reynolds CF 3rd, Butters MA, Lopez O, et al. Maintenance treatment of depression in old age: a randomized, double-blind, placebo-controlled evaluation of the efficacy and safety of donepezil combined with antidepressant pharmacotherapy. Arch Gen Psychiatry 2011;68(1):51–60.

109. Richard E, Reitz C, Honig LH, et al. Late-life depression, mild cognitive impairment, and dementia. JAMA Neurol 2013;70(3):374–82.

Dealing with Mild Cognitive Impairment
Help for Patients and Caregivers

Donald L. Courtney, MD

KEYWORDS

- Mild cognitive impairment • Alzheimer disease • Activities of daily living
- Dementia progression • Cognitive training

KEY POINTS

- Patients diagnosed with MCI face an uncertain future, with some progressing to develop dementia. Helping patients and families cope is important in managing MCI.
- Families need to know signs of progression to dementia, including loss of independence of activities of daily living or impaired social functioning.
- Optimal management of comorbid illnesses may provide improved cognition; these may be permanent.
- Physical exercise, specific brain exercises, and dietary factors are associated with improvements in cognition in healthy elderly, and may be effective in MCI.

INTRODUCTION

Mild cognitive impairment (MCI) is a unique entity in the spectrum of syndromes of cognitive loss. Most patients who present with preserved activities of daily living (ADLs) and a noticeable decline in cognitive ability have MCI. Amnestic MCI involves memory as the principal loss, and new learning is the most impaired part of memory. When discussing patient and family needs, within this article, the focus is on amnestic MCI.

Many patients referred for evaluation of memory loss come with an assumption that they already have dementia. The patient or caregiver has expressed concerns about memory loss, the primary care provider has done a screening test and has found deficits, and the patients hear or infer that they have dementia. One of the biggest challenges is to offer the patient reassurance that they are "not yet demented, and may never develop dementia," tempered with the need to discuss planning for the real possibility that they have a 35% to 40% chance of developing dementia in the next 4 years.

Funding Sources: None.
Conflict of Interest: None.
Section of Geriatric Medicine (11G), Division of General and Geriatric Medicine, Department of Medicine, Ralph H. Johnson VA Medical Center, Medical University of South Carolina, 109 Bee Street, Charleston, SC 29401, USA
E-mail address: Donald.Courtney2@va.gov

When a patient is diagnosed with MCI, the patient and caregivers alike have to deal with the challenge of uncertainties. The spectrum of MCI can encompass patients with very early Alzheimer disease who will progress in their cognitive impairment over the next few years; it also can include a more benign syndrome of patients with stable cognitive deficits over several years, and a small number of patients who actually improve on repeated cognitive testing in future years.

Significant promise exists that specialized testing will be able to separate the more benign MCI syndromes from early Alzheimer disease. At present, the tests are not sufficiently established to be predictive, are not clinically available outside of research sites, and/or are not reimbursed by most insurance providers. Other articles in this issue outline the diagnosis and current stage of research regarding biomarkers and imaging studies. This article is written with the purpose of guiding the clinician who has reached a diagnosis of MCI, and is working with the patient and family on coping with the uncertainties of MCI.

Patient and family education has to stress the uncertainty of whether the deficits will progress, warning signs, coping strategies for now and the future, and full discussions of advanced directives while the patient is still able to make decisions. The clinician needs to offer the patient and family an overarching philosophy of "hope for the best; prepare for the worst."

WILL THE PATIENT GET WORSE?

Possibly. The risk of progressing to dementia is about 15% per year for the next 3 or 4 years, with the risk in later years unknown. Many patients will remain stable for over a decade.

WHAT ARE THE WARNING SIGNS THE PATIENT AND FAMILY SHOULD LOOK FOR THAT INDICATE THE PATIENT IS GETTING WORSE?

When memory problems interfere with the patient's ability to perform ADLs, it is an undeniable sign of progression. Examples include needing help with selecting clothes or dressing, or needing assistance with bathing or hygiene.

Less certain signs that the disease is progressing include difficulty with cooking familiar dishes, performing usual housekeeping chores, money management, and driving familiar routes. Family members of patients with MCI need to oversee the bill-paying on a monthly or every-other-month basis, to make certain that important bills are being paid on time.

Personality changes may be a sign of worsening disease. Outbursts of anger, withdrawal from usual activities, neglect of hygiene, and decreased social interaction may all be signs of progression to dementia.

Depression occurs with some frequency in early dementia and in MCI; the concentration difficulty and personality changes may not be signs of progression of dementia, but treatable depression. As discussed later, regular annual screening for depression in patients with MCI, coupled with treatment of the depression, may improve the patient's memory and independence.

HOW CAN PATIENTS IMPROVE THEIR MEMORY, OR SLOW ITS DECLINE?

It should be obvious that other medical conditions should be optimally treated. Three in particular have solid evidence that proper treatment improves cognitive function: obstructive sleep apnea (OSA), obesity, and diabetes.

Obstructive Sleep Apnea

OSA increases in frequency with aging. It is associated with problems in concentration, attention, and memory. In a prospective study of community-living cognitively intact women who underwent sleep studies, those with sleep-disordered breathing were 85% more likely to develop MCI or dementia over a 4-year follow-up than those without sleep-disordered breathing.[1]

If untreated OSA puts patients at risk for MCI or dementia, then does treatment improve cognition? In an interventional study of continuous positive airway pressure (CPAP), placebo-CPAP, or supplemental oxygen treatment in patients with OSA,[2] subjects underwent neuropsychiatric testing before treatment and after 2 weeks of CPAP treatment. Before treatment, patients with OSA showed diffuse impairments, particularly in terms of speed of information processing, attention and working memory, executive functioning, learning and memory, as well as alertness and sustained attention. Modest improvements were seen after 2 weeks of CPAP in comparison with the group that received supplemental oxygen or placebo-CPAP. The investigators concluded that "2 weeks of CPAP treatment might be helpful in terms of speed of information processing, vigilance, or sustained attention and alertness." It is possible that further benefits might be seen over longer periods of treatment.

Obesity

Obesity is associated with cognitive loss. Recent twin studies[3] on middle-aged obesity shows obesity itself to be an independent predictor of both cardiovascular disease and cognitive decline in old age. Of note, a recent meta-analysis[4] of studies of intentional weight loss found improvements in memory and attention with weight loss.

Diabetes Mellitus

Diabetes is associated with an increased risk of cognitive loss with aging. Studies looking at this relationship have found that there are more strokes in persons with diabetes, which is thought to be responsible for much of the increased risk of cognitive loss seen in diabetes. Important for the discussion of MCI is that diabetics with poor control (higher levels of glycosylated hemoglobin) showed more decline in cognition over a 9-year study, independent of cerebrovascular disease.[5] Good diabetes control appears to protect patients from cognitive loss.

Although weight loss and diabetes control have not been specifically studied in subjects with MCI, it is reasonable at present to recommend weight loss and good diabetes control for their global benefits, with a reasonable expectation that they will have a positive impact on cognition.

Other Interventions

Beyond managing other diseases, there are several interventions that may help patients with MCI to improve or maintain function. Patients and families will find claims of benefit for various products. Patients should be encouraged to check out any claims against the National Institutes of Health clinical trials registry to find out whether the product has demonstrated any effects on memory. In May 2013, there were 376 registered studies on MCI, including interventions with drugs, dietary supplements, mental exercise, and physical exercise.

Drugs

At present, there are no medications approved by the Food and Drug Administration for MCI. Specifically, the drugs approved for dementia (cholinesterase inhibitors, memantine) have been studied and have not been found to be effective in treating MCI.

Diet and nutrition

Several nutritional supplements/nutraceuticals claim to improve memory, but there are none with specific data regarding MCI that show improvement.

The author's group is currently involved in studies of micronutrients that stimulate nerve differentiation in an animal model of Alzheimer disease, and are enrolling subjects with MCI for longitudinal studies of cognitive function and biomarkers of Alzheimer disease.

A multivitamin with generous amounts of antioxidants is a safe treatment that may offer as much protection against cognitive decline as more expensive high-dose therapies. High-dose vitamin E,[6] and usual doses of vitamin D for prevention of bone loss,[7] have not been shown to be effective in MCI. A longitudinal study of 107 dietary items in Australia found an association between diets highest in processed foods and MCI[8]; a recommendation for more fresh fruits and vegetables seems reasonable for several health-related reasons, which now include a possible benefit to memory.

Physical exercise

There is growing evidence of a link between physical activity and improved cognitive function in patients with MCI. A recent study of a multicomponent exercise program (aerobic exercise, strength training, postural balance training, totaling to 180 minutes per week for 12 months) found small improvements in Mini Mental Status Examination (MMSE) scores, immediate recall, and verbal fluency.[9] Population-based studies have found that elderly subjects who report participating in regular physical exercise were less likely to develop MCI.[10] Of note, subjects who participated in regular physical exercise and were engaged in computer use had a 64% reduction in likelihood of developing MCI when compared with subjects who were neither exercisers nor computer users.

Brain exercises

Patients and families need to know that the brain with MCI may still be capable of new learning. It is reasonable to encourage patients to try to exercise their brain to improve their ability to function. Most patients are eager to try these interventions; there are limited data on persistence outside of a small number of clinical trials.

There is significant interest in brain training at present, with at least 3 popular computer-based brain-training programs being marketed to the elderly in general, or specifically to patients with MCI (Lumosity.com, Cognifit.com, Positscience.com). Patients and families need to be aware that although some benefits are seen with brain training, we do not have a full understanding of what these benefits may be. The comparative benefits of different brain-training programs, and the best way to improve function for individuals with particular deficits, remain unknown.

One study of computer-based cognitive training in subjects older than 65 years without a diagnosis of clinically significant cognitive impairment (normal elderly) found improvements in several domains of neuropsychological testing after training, which weakened in 3 months without training.[11] The ACTIVE (Advanced Cognitive Training for Independent and Vital Elderly) study of computer-based brain training had a 10-session initial phase, with booster training offered to participants at 11 and 35 months. There were 3 different training interventions (memory, reasoning, speed of processing), plus a control group. The subjects in the speed-of-processing group had significant improvements in self-rated health at 2, 3, and 5-year follow-up.[12]

Speed-of-processing brain training may also be effective in maintaining independence. Slower mental processing has been identified as a risk factor that leads older patients to stop driving.[13] Computer-based speed-of-processing training was provided to half of a cohort of 550 subjects; the exercises of visual attention were designed to target speed and accuracy of visual performance. Ten sessions were provided, with 88% of subjects in the treatment group receiving all 10 sessions. At the end of 3 years of follow-up, subjects who underwent training were 40% less likely to give up driving than subjects in the control group (9% vs 14%).[14] Subjects in this study had MMSE scores of 23 or better; there was no specific diagnosis of MCI. One cohort of subjects[15] for this study was a group with a poor useful field of view (UFOV). Though not correlated with other markers of cognitive decline, decreased UFOV may be more prevalent in patients with MCI.

At Stanford, Rosen and colleagues[16] have demonstrated that specific training to improve verbal memory, compared with a control group that performed other computer activities, resulted in significantly improved verbal memory scores. In addition to improved test scores, subjects who received verbal memory training had increased activity on functional magnetic resonance imaging (MRI) in the left hippocampus (the hippocampus is one of the earliest sites where changes specific to Alzheimer disease are seen). The investigators suggest that the hippocampus in MCI may retain sufficient neuroplasticity to benefit from cognitive training. This study, with the combination of control groups, cognitive improvement on specific neuropsychological testing, and corresponding changes in functional MRI, provides some of the best evidence that brain training in the early stages of MCI can be effective.

If patients are interested in brain training, they should be encouraged to identify a program that includes speed-of-processing drills, and to stick with the program as long as they can. Patients understand the analogy to muscle training: there are many ways to exercise muscles, some produce more obvious benefits than do others, and benefits tend to disappear after the training stops.

ARE THERE FACTORS THAT MIGHT MAKE COGNITION WORSE?

There is little evidence that the progression of amnestic MCI is accelerated by specific events. The following concerns are based on conditions that aggravate dementia; it is plausible that they have similar impacts on MCI.

Drugs

Several classes of medications can worsen dementia. The clinician should try to stop any of these drugs in patients with memory deficits, whether they score as MCI or dementia.

Drugs with anticholinergic effects are well-described causes of decreased memory. Given the depletion of acetylcholine in the brains of patients with Alzheimer disease, the connection makes sense. Anticholinergic drugs are common, with uses for diarrhea, urinary urgency, some of the symptoms of Parkinson disease, and some of the side effects of antipsychotic drugs. Many other drugs have anticholinergic effects. **Table 1**[17] lists drugs to avoid.

Other drugs to avoid include sedatives and opiates, given the frequency of clouding consciousness and decreasing alertness. The caveat is that with better pain control from an opiate, some patients sleep better and are more awake and alert. A therapeutic trial is the only way to be confirm this proposal.

Over-the-counter medications are sometimes influential. It is important to ask about cold remedies, sleeping aids, and alcohol-based cough syrups.

Alcohol use should be reviewed, and moderate use to abstinence should be strongly recommended.

Table 1 Drugs to avoid in MCI		
High Anticholinergic Activity	Moderate Anticholinergic Activity	Low Anticholinergic Activity
Amitriptyline	Chlorpromazine	Cimetidine
Benztropine	Darifenacin	Citalopram
Clozapine	Desipramine	Escitalopram
Cyclobenzaprine	Diphenhydramine	Fluoxetine
Dicyclomine	Disopyramide	Haloperidol
Doxepin	Fesoterodine	Lithium
L-Hyosciamine	Hydroxyzine	Mirtazapine
Scopolamine	Nortriptyline	Quetiapine
Thioridazine	Olanzapine	Ranitidine
Trihexyphenidyl	Oxybutynin	Temazepam
	Paroxetine	
	Solifenacin	
	Tolterodine	
	Trospium	
	Venlafaxine	

Hospitalization

Hospitalization in older adults, with and without baseline cognitive impairment, is often associated with cognitive loss. In most cases, cognition returns to prehospital baseline within a few weeks. Separating the effect of the acute disease that prompted hospitalization from the disorienting routine of the hospital is not possible. The importance of this risk factor concerns provider and family awareness. The frequent answer to the question: "When did you first notice your parent's thinking was impaired?" is "Right after surgery," or "When she was hospitalized with chest pain." Investigators believe there is a preclinical phase of dementia during which the brain is losing reserve but is not yet noticeably impaired. The stress of illness, medications, a new environment and routine, and sleep deprivation may produce acute delirium. It is not clear how commonly an episode of delirium predicts MCI or dementia, but some correlation is apparent.

Depression

All patients with MCI need to be screened for depression. Cognitive changes in the depressed elderly include impaired memory, delayed processing, and decreased attention. Treatment of depression may reverse some or all cognitive changes.

HOW CAN CLINICIANS HELP PATIENTS PLAN FOR THE FUTURE?

Patients with MCI should complete as much planning as possible so as to prepare for a time when they cannot make decisions. The planning needed extends far beyond the medical model. Several well-written books can be used as resources for patient and family teaching, and planning for the future.

How Can Patients Prepare an Advanced Directive that Would Span Several Years, When Their Goals Will Likely Change as they Lose Independence?

When time is available, a discussion about advanced directives and medical decisions should take place, focusing on the goals of health care.[18] In summary, health care serves 3 purposes: prolonging life, maximizing cognitive and functional independence, and relieving suffering. Whenever possible, interventions that accomplish all 3 goals are selected. As a patient's disease becomes more advanced, cure becomes impossible, and life expectancy decreases, the importance of those 3 different goals changes. In most chronic diseases, and with advancing age, patients and caregivers have to select which goal is most important, and allow that goal to determine the specific treatments. The Venn diagram of 3 overlapping circles is an effective way of communicating this concept. When there no treatment available that is expected to prolong life, maximize independence, and relieve suffering, patients and families have to choose treatments most consistent with the stated goals of care.

After understanding this concept, patients and their families often make a declaration about changing their goals of care based on anticipated landmarks in cognitive or functional loss. Examples include:

- "If my wife is embarrassed to take me out in public, I don't want to do anything to keep me alive longer."
- "If our money is being depleted to keep me in a nursing home, I don't want to do anything to make me live longer."
- "If I can't control my bowels, just keep me comfortable and don't do anything to prolong my life in that condition."
- "If I can't feed myself, I don't want a feeding tube."

Patients need to discuss these situations with their family. If there is a clear understanding by both, they should write down the agreement and sign it. These "If..., then" statements are a useful start to the idea of changing treatment goals as a patient's condition changes.

The next phase is a more global one: to make global judgments about the effectiveness of interventions to meet different goals, and make decisions about cardiopulmonary resuscitation (CPR), stays in the intensive care unit (ICU), surgical treatment, or hospitalization. For example, when prolonging life is no longer the most important goal, CPR is not indicated. Even if it is successful there is likely to be a period of time in the ICU, and if the patient survives beyond the ICU, functional decline is almost certain. Patients and caregivers can appreciate the idea of selecting different goals of care as diseases progress, and letting those goals determine specific interventions. **Table 2** summarizes the changing importance of these goals, and the decisions that follow.

Some patients and families are able to make decisions using these pathways, and suggest discrete points in the course of their illness at which they would want to change goals, usually at times of loss of independence.

One of the advantages of having a patient select one of the pathways listed is that it gives a framework for the family to decide about an intervention that was not discussed. The patient and family can discuss with the caregiver if the intervention has a high likelihood of meeting the most important goal. If not, an alternative treatment may be the better option.

Decisions about artificial feedings are among the most difficult for caregivers.[19] Patients need to decide now, at the stage of MCI, if they would want a feeding tube if they become dependent to the point they cannot swallow, presenting information about the lack of efficacy of tube feedings to prevent pneumonia or death,[20] and the greater than 70% rate of use of restraint to prevent dementia patients from trying to remove the tube.[21] The thought of being tied down to have nutrients pumped into their abdomen is probably the most difficult scenario for patients to imagine as they discuss advanced directives. All of the patients in the author's experience to date have explicitly wished not to have tube feedings if they lose the ability to swallow safely.

Table 2
Changing importance of goals, and the decisions that follow

Title	Most Important	Second Most Important	Least Important	Interventions
Intensive pathway	Living as long as possible	Being as independent as possible	Not suffering	All medically indicated procedures, including CPR, ventilator support, ICU care
Comprehensive pathway	Being as independent as possible	Living as long as possible	Not suffering	CPR and ICU care are rarely indicated
Basic pathway	Being as independent as possible	Not suffering	Living as long as possible	Outpatient care for as much as possible, surgery only indicated where independence is likely to increase (eg, repair of hip fracture)
Palliative pathway	Not suffering	Being as independent as possible	Living as long as possible	Strictly home care or nursing home care, minimal diagnostic tests
Comfort-only pathway	Not suffering is the only goal	—	—	Treatment is exclusively to relieve symptoms; pneumonia would be treated with oxygen and morphine for the air hunger, not with antibiotics

Abbreviations: CPR, cardiopulmonary resuscitation; ICU, intensive care unit.

When Should an Older Person with MCI or Early Dementia Stop Driving?

Clinicians have recommended using the phrase "retire from driving" to introduce the subject. The analogy that a person retires from a job seems to change the mindset about continuing to drive.[22] There are very few rules or medical criteria to guide when to stop driving. Drivers' insight into their own ability has been poor, whether there are memory problems or not.[23] The AARP (formerly the American Association of Retired Persons) offers a program on driving safety for the elderly that offers general advice on safer driving (which is not specific to cognitive loss, but does deal with the slower reaction times of aging). Patients should be encouraged to participate in a class if they intend to continue driving.

Physicians are asked to screen older patients for driving safety. At conflict is the desire to preserve the independence of the patient while protecting others.[24] Balancing the risk/benefit of these two competing interests is difficult. One technique to guide the clinician on when to advise the patient to stop driving is to ask the caregiver: "If the two of you are going someplace together, are you willing to ride in the car and let them drive?" Many children of patients will initially want the older person to continue to drive and stay independent, but admit they feel unsafe riding with the patient at the wheel. If the family does not feel safe riding with the patient driving, the patient needs to retire from driving.

Should Firearms be Removed from the House?

Some groups have advocated removing guns from the house of patients with dementia, and the question then becomes: "At what point in cognitive loss should the guns be removed?" There are no data on this subject. There is no evidence that patients with amnestic MCI are at any special risk for gun-related issues. However, the patient with personality changes (eg, anger outbursts), the patient who expresses paranoid ideations ("my husband is having an affair."), or the patient with hallucinations has an increased potential for unpredictable violence. In these cases, the patients have crossed the line from MCI to dementia. When patients exhibit 1 of these personality or thought disorders the house needs to be made safe, with guns removed and only knives needed for cooking kept in the house.

WHAT INTERVENTIONS ARE THERE FOR THE CAREGIVER?

Information about community resources is the most important intervention for the caregiver. Caregivers should contact the local chapter of the Alzheimer's Association (www.alz.org). The caregiver can find resources, support classes, and activities for grassroots involvement and activism at the Alzheimer's Association. The Area Agency on Aging in their county will have information about local resources as well. Knowing that adult day care is available, even if not used, is reassuring for caregivers.

Many families are interested in identifying potential treatments as soon as possible. As mentioned earlier, caregivers should check out www.clinicaltrials.com regularly, searching for "mild cognitive impairment." Caregivers may be able to find information about trials in their area; they can see what interventions have been studied and where study results are available, and if the interventions have shown benefit. Caregivers can also identify local experts in the disease if such experts are conducting clinical research.

Task Simplification

With impaired memory, apparently simple tasks become too complex. An effective strategy for the caregiver is to break a complex task into a series of simple tasks. Setting the table is a useful example: if a patient cannot set the table, change the request. The caregiver should instead ask the patient to "put two plates on the table where we sit to eat"; then ask him or her to get napkins and put them beside the plates; then silverware; then glasses filled with water. The memory-impaired patient is able to contribute more to chores around the house, working within preserved mental capacity.

Memory Aids

Patients and caregivers need to write things down. MCI patients should get into the habit of keeping a small notebook and pen in their pocket as they go through the day. If they start this habit early in MCI, it may help them through progressive memory loss.

In addition to old-fashioned pen and paper, there is interest in using smartphones (or PDAs) to assist patients with MCI. At Toronto, Svoboda's group[25] has published positive studies over the last 6 years, with significant improvement in global function and specific tasks.

Families can be encouraged to buy a smartphone for the patient, and to activate the GPS tracking function. The GPS tracking will be useful if the phone is lost, but also if the MCI patient who progresses to dementia wanders away from home but remembers to take the phone. It has the potential, if it becomes a habit to always carry it, to have benefit in early MCI and in later stages of dementia.

SUMMARY

MCI is a difficult disease for patients and caregivers. The uncertainty of prognosis hangs over the patient and caregiver, up to the point at which they develop dementia. Because some patients never progress as far as dementia, they live the rest of their lives with uncertainty. As much as the uncertainty is frustrating to patients and family, it is better to persist in MCI and be uncertain about next year than to watch the patient progress to dementia. Patients and families should be encouraged to do as much as possible to work within their MCI, building on their strengths. Physical exercise, brain training, and planning for possible progression are important interventions for this disease of uncertainty.

Effective treatment is not known. There is benefit from managing other diseases well, especially sleep apnea, obesity, and diabetes. There are benefits from eating healthily, physical exercise, and mental exercises. Specific mental exercise programs are as yet not well known.

Avoiding drugs that can affect cognition is important. Specific guidance about alcohol use does not exist, but low use to abstinence seems prudent. Avoiding high-stress environments such as hospitals is beneficial, although hospital care is beneficial for concurrent illness.

Patients and families need to "hope for the best, and prepare for the worst." Patients should be encouraged to engage in discussions and written instructions for their wishes to be met, and be offered a framework for altering wishes as cognitive loss progresses.

Caregiver support becomes important if dementia progresses; families need to make contact with the local Alzheimer's Association early on. Memory aids may be helpful for patients coping with memory loss. There is promise that smartphones may help patients compensate for memory loss, but training of patients with MCI in the use of the smartphone requires several sessions.

REFERENCES

1. Yaffe K, Laffan AM, Harrison SL, et al. Sleep-disordered breathing, hypoxia, and risk of mild cognitive impairment and dementia in older women. JAMA 2011; 306(6):613–9.
2. Lim W, Bardwell WA, Loredo JS, et al. Neuropsychological effects of 2 week continuous positive airway pressure treatment and supplemental oxygen in patients with obstructive sleep apnea: a randomized, placebo-controlled study. J Clin Sleep Med 2007;3(4):380–6.
3. Laitala VS, Kaprio J, Koskenvuo M, et al. Association and causal relationship of midlife obesity and related metabolic disorders with old age cognition. Curr Alzheimer Res 2011;8(6):699–706.
4. Siervo M, Arnold R, Wells JC, et al. Intentional weight loss in overweight and obese individuals and cognitive function: a systematic review and meta-analysis. Obes Rev 2011;12(11):968–83.
5. Yaffe K, Falvey C, Hamilton N, et al. Diabetes, glucose control, and 9-year cognitive decline among older adults without dementia. Arch Neurol 2012;69(9): 1170–5.
6. Farina N, Isaac MG, Clark AR, et al. Vitamin E for Alzheimer's dementia and mild cognitive impairment. Cochrane Database Syst Rev 2012;(11):CD002854.

7. Rossom RC, Espeland MA, Manson JE, et al. Calcium and vitamin D supplementation and cognitive impairment in the Women's Health Initiative. J Am Geriatr Soc 2012;60(12):2197–205.
8. Torres SJ, Lautenschlager NT, Wattanapenpaiboon M, et al. Dietary patterns are associated with cognition among older people with mild cognitive impairment. Nutrients 2012;4(11):1542–51.
9. Suzuki T, Shimada H, Makizako H, et al. Effects of multicomponent exercise on cognitive function in WMS-LM older adults with amnestic mild cognitive impairment: a randomized controlled trial. BMC Neurol 2012;12(1):128.
10. Geda YE, Silber TC, Roberts RO, et al. Computer activities, physical exercise, aging and mild cognitive impairment: a population-based study. Mayo Clin Proc 2012;87(5):437–42.
11. Zelinski EM, Spina LM, Yaffe K, et al. Improvement in memory with plasticity-based adaptive cognitive training: results of the 3-month follow-up. J Am Geriatr Soc 2011;59(2):258–65.
12. Wolinsky FD, Mahncke H, Vander Weg MW, et al. Speed of processing training protects self-rated health in older adults: enduring effects observed in the multi-site ACTIVE randomized controlled trial. Int Psychogeriatr 2010;22(3):470–8.
13. Edwards JD, Ross LA, Ackerman ML, et al. Longitudinal predictors of driving cessation among older adults from the ACTIVE clinical trial. J Gerontol B Psychol Sci Soc Sci 2008;63(1):P6–12.
14. Edwards JD, Delahunt PB, Mahncke HW. Cognitive speed of processing training delays driving cessation. J Gerontol A Biol Sci Med Sci 2009;64(12):1262–7.
15. Edwards JD, Myers C, Ross LA, et al. The longitudinal impact of cognitive speed of processing training on driving mobility. Gerontologist 2009;49(4):485–94.
16. Rosen AC, Sugiura L, Kramer JH, et al. Cognitive training changes hippocampal function in mild cognitive impairment: a pilot study. J Alzheimers Dis 2011; 26(Suppl 3):349–57.
17. Reuben DB, Herr KA, Pacala HT, et al. Geriatrics at your fingertips: 2012. 14th edition. New York: The American Geriatrics Society; 2012.
18. Gillick M, Berkman S, Cullen L. A patient-centered approach to advance medical planning in the nursing home. J Am Geriatr Soc 1999;47(2):227–30.
19. Rabins PV, Hicks KL, Black BS. Medical decisions made by surrogates for persons with advanced dementia within weeks or months of death. AJOB Prim Res 2011;2(4):61–5.
20. Finucane TE, Christmas C, Travis K. Tube feedings in patients with advanced dementia: a review of the evidence. JAMA 1999;282(14):1365–70.
21. Peck A, Cohen CE, Mulvihill MN. Long-term enteral feeding of aged demented nursing home patients. J Am Geriatr Soc 1990;38(11):1195–8.
22. Mizuno Y, Arai Y. Measures to support voluntary retirement from driving in Japanese older people: driving is not just a means of transportation. J Am Geriatr Soc 2012;60(11):2170–2.
23. Sevensen O. Are we all less risky and more skillful than our fellow drivers? Acta Psychol (Amst) 1981;47(2):143–8.
24. Graca J. Driving and aging. Clin Geriatr Med 1986;2(3):577–89.
25. Svoboda E, Richards B, Leach L, et al. PDA and smartphone use by individuals with moderate-to-severe memory impairment: application of a theory-driven training programme. Neuropsychol Rehabil 2012;22(3):408–27.

Index

Clin Geriatr Med 29 (2013) 907–913
http://dx.doi.org/10.1016/S0749-0690(13)00075-X
0749-0690/13/$ – see front matter © 2013 Elsevier Inc. All rights reserved.

geriatric.theclinics.com

United States Postal Service
Statement of Ownership, Management, and Circulation
(All Periodicals Publications Except Requestor Publications)

1. Publication Title	2. Publication Number	3. Filing Date
Clinics in Geriatric Medicine	0 0 0 - 7 0 4	9/14/13

4. Issue Frequency	5. Number of Issues Published Annually	6. Annual Subscription Price
Feb, May, Aug, Nov	4	$269.00

7. Complete Mailing Address of Known Office of Publication (Not printer) (Street, city, county, state, and ZIP+4®)

Elsevier Inc.
360 Park Avenue South
New York, NY 10010-1710

Contact Person: Stephen R. Bushing

Telephone (Include area code): 215-239-3688

8. Complete Mailing Address of Headquarters or General Business Office of Publisher (Not printer)

Elsevier Inc., 360 Park Avenue South, New York, NY 10010-1710

9. Full Names and Complete Mailing Addresses of Publisher, Editor, and Managing Editor (Do not leave blank)

Publisher (Name and complete mailing address)

Linda Belfus, Elsevier, Inc., 1600 John F. Kennedy Blvd. Suite 1800, Philadelphia, PA 19103-2899

Editor (Name and complete mailing address)

Yonah Korngold, Elsevier, Inc., 1600 John F. Kennedy Blvd. Suite 1800, Philadelphia, PA 19103-2899

Managing Editor (Name and complete mailing address)

Barbara Cohen - Kligerman, Elsevier, Inc., 1600 John F. Kennedy Blvd. Suite 1800, Philadelphia, PA 19103-2899

10. Owner (Do not leave blank. If the publication is owned by a corporation, give the name and address of the corporation immediately followed by the names and addresses of all stockholders owning or holding 1 percent or more of the total amount of stock. If not owned by a corporation, give the names and addresses of the individual owners. If owned by a partnership or other unincorporated firm, give its name and address as well as those of each individual owner. If the publication is published by a nonprofit organization, give its name and address.)

Full Name	Complete Mailing Address
Wholly owned subsidiary of	1600 John F. Kennedy Blvd., Ste. 1800
Reed/Elsevier, US holdings	Philadelphia, PA 19103-2899

11. Known Bondholders, Mortgagees, and Other Security Holders Owning or Holding 1 Percent or More of Total Amount of Bonds, Mortgages, or Other Securities. If none, check box ☐ None

Full Name	Complete Mailing Address
N/A	

12. Tax Status (For completion by nonprofit organizations authorized to mail at nonprofit rates) (Check one)
The purpose, function, and nonprofit status of this organization and the exempt status for federal income tax purposes:
☐ Has Not Changed During Preceding 12 Months
☐ Has Changed During Preceding 12 Months (Publisher must submit explanation of change with this statement)

PS Form 3526, September 2007 (Page 1 of 3 (Instructions Page 3)) PSN 7530-01-000-9931 PRIVACY NOTICE: See our Privacy policy in www.usps.com

---

13. Publication Title	14. Issue Date for Circulation Data Below
Clinics in Geriatric Medicine	August 2013

15.	Extent and Nature of Circulation		Average No. Copies Each Issue During Preceding 12 Months	No. Copies of Single Issue Published Nearest to Filing Date
a.	Total Number of Copies (Net press run)		539	443
b. Paid Circulation (By Mail and Outside the Mail)	(1)	Mailed Outside-County Paid Subscriptions Stated on PS Form 3541. (Include paid distribution above nominal rate, advertiser's proof copies, and exchange copies)	277	239
	(2)	Mailed In-County Paid Subscriptions Stated on PS Form 3541 (Include paid distribution above nominal rate, advertiser's proof copies, and exchange copies)		
	(3)	Paid Distribution Outside the Mails Including Sales Through Dealers and Carriers, Street Vendors, Counter Sales, and Other Paid Distribution Outside USPS®	107	89
	(4)	Paid Distribution by Other Classes Mailed Through the USPS (e.g. First-Class Mail®)		
c.	Total Paid Distribution (Sum of 15b (1), (2), (3), and (4)) ▲		384	328
d. Free or Nominal Rate Distribution (By Mail and Outside the Mail)	(1)	Free or Nominal Rate Outside-County Copies Included on PS Form 3541	60	64
	(2)	Free or Nominal Rate In-County Copies Included on PS Form 3541		
	(3)	Free or Nominal Rate Copies Mailed at Other Classes Through the USPS (e.g. First-Class Mail)		
	(4)	Free or Nominal Rate Distribution Outside the Mail (Carriers or other means)		
e.	Total Free or Nominal Rate Distribution (Sum of 15d (1), (2), (3) and (4)) ▲		60	64
f.	Total Distribution (Sum of 15c and 15e) ▲		444	392
g.	Copies not Distributed (See instructions to publishers #4 (page #3)) ▲		95	51
h.	Total (Sum of 15f and g) ▲		539	443
i.	Percent Paid (15c divided by 15f times 100)		86.49%	83.67%

16. Publication of Statement of Ownership
☐ If the publication is a general publication, publication of this statement is required. Will be printed in the November 2013 issue of this publication. ☐ Publication not required

17. Signature and Title of Editor, Publisher, Business Manager, or Owner	Date
[signature] Stephen R. Bushing – Inventory Distribution Coordinator	September 14, 2013

I certify that all information furnished on this form is true and complete. I understand that anyone who furnishes false or misleading information on this form or who omits material or information requested on the form may be subject to criminal sanctions (including fines and imprisonment) and/or civil sanctions (including civil penalties).

PS Form 3526, September 2007 (Page 2 of 3)

Moving?

Make sure your subscription moves with you!

To notify us of your new address, find your **Clinics Account Number** (located on your mailing label above your name), and contact customer service at:

Email: journalscustomerservice-usa@elsevier.com

800-654-2452 (subscribers in the U.S. & Canada)
314-447-8871 (subscribers outside of the U.S. & Canada)

Fax number: 314-447-8029

Elsevier Health Sciences Division
Subscription Customer Service
3251 Riverport Lane
Maryland Heights, MO 63043

*To ensure uninterrupted delivery of your subscription, please notify us at least 4 weeks in advance of move.

Printed and bound by CPI Group (UK) Ltd, Croydon, CR0 4YY

03/10/2024

01040493-0016